Also by Alisha Gaddis

Your House Keys are in the Dryer:
A Parenting Haiku Book

PERIODS,
PERIOD.

WRITTEN BY ALISHA GADDIS & STEPH GARCIA

Post Hill
PRESS

A POST HILL PRESS BOOK
ISBN: 978-1-63758-554-2
ISBN (eBook): 978-1-63758-555-9

Periods, Period.
© 2023 by Alisha Gaddis & Steph Garcia
All Rights Reserved

Illustrations by Desireé Nash
Cover design by Tiffani Shea

Post Hill Press
New York • Nashville
posthillpress.com

Published in the United States of America

1 2 3 4 5 6 7 8 9 10

Periods, Period. is a book for entertainment purposes only. We hope that it begins you on your menstruation info journey and makes you laugh along the way. Please always consult medical professionals if you have any concerns regarding your period and/or your body.

FOREWORD

There are fantastic books out there that focus on the anatomical and physical changes that happen once you have your period. We highly recommend reading those to get more understanding of what goes on inside your body during puberty and menstruation.

Because this is not that book.

This book was put together as a fun way to look at your period because there's a lot to laugh at and a lot to connect over. Menstruation happens to a large swath of the human population (and let's be real, a lot of other animals as well). So, let's stop making it feel so secret! Or taboo!

Feel free to jump around within these pages and land on whatever will make you feel good while you're bleeding. Sync your period with your BFF and do some of the pages together! Highlight, take notes, write in the specifics about your experience—so you can not only better know your period but know you're not alone in this menstruation journey.

Let's bleed together! Bleed loudly, quietly, boldly, laughingly.

Let it bleed!

WHAT TO EXPECT ON YOUR PERIOD...

EVERYTHING.

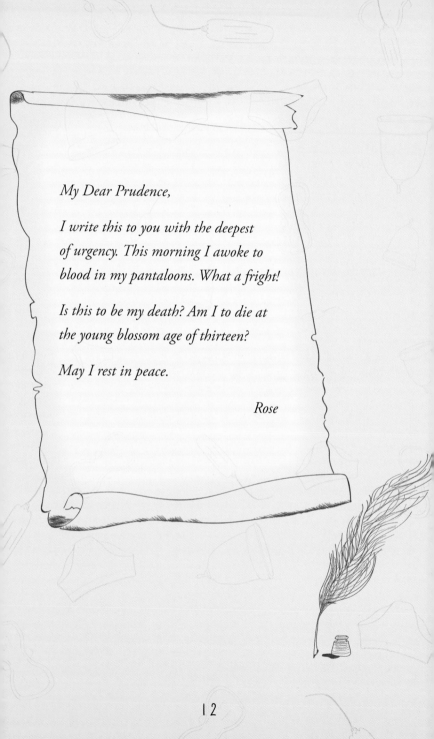

My Dear Prudence,

I write this to you with the deepest of urgency. This morning I awoke to blood in my pantaloons. What a fright!

Is this to be my death? Am I to die at the young blossom age of thirteen?

May I rest in peace.

Rose

Dearest Rose,

The mail came today. Imagine my delight to see a letter from you! I would have never imagined the intensity of experience that burst forth through your words.

This happens every month, I am told! Bleeding every month? Can you imagine, Rose?

Be not fearful. You shall survive.

Prudence

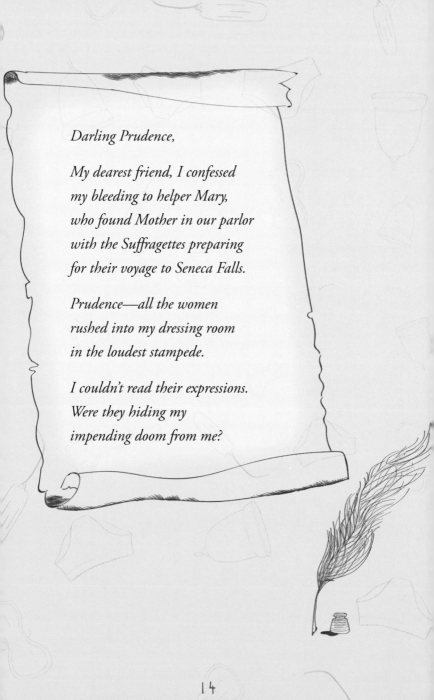

Darling Prudence,

*My dearest friend, I confessed
my bleeding to helper Mary,
who found Mother in our parlor
with the Suffragettes preparing
for their voyage to Seneca Falls.*

*Prudence—all the women
rushed into my dressing room
in the loudest stampede.*

*I couldn't read their expressions.
Were they hiding my
impending doom from me?*

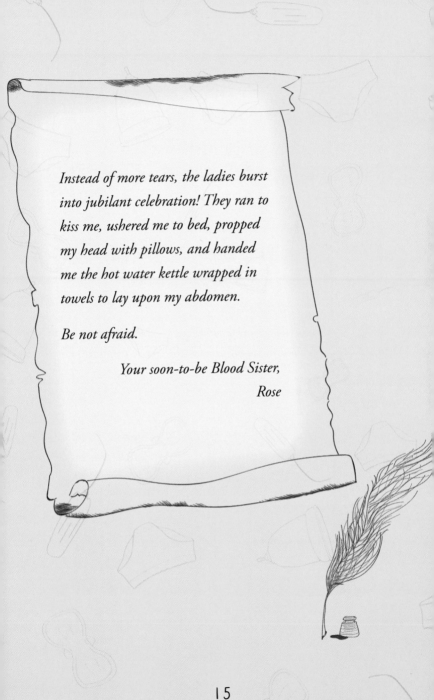

Instead of more tears, the ladies burst into jubilant celebration! They ran to kiss me, ushered me to bed, propped my head with pillows, and handed me the hot water kettle wrapped in towels to lay upon my abdomen.

Be not afraid.

Your soon-to-be Blood Sister,
Rose

Dearest Rose,

I shall be checking my bedsheets every morning for the bright red intruder!

You have instilled courage in me for this next chapter in our lives—bleeding out monthly. I know it will come. Our cat, Harriet, was in heat this summer. What a time to remember!

I only wish we were closer and could share our menses in misery together.

Waiting for the blood to drop,

Prudence

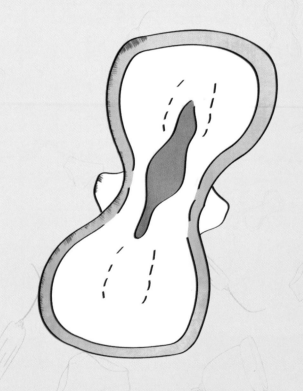

MYDOLLHOUSE

Welcome to the Home of Period Self-Care:

The MYDOLL House

All the feelings. All the feelings. ALL THE FEELINGS.

Rest, recover, relish.

Emote, hide out, find yourself.

All the things, in your house.

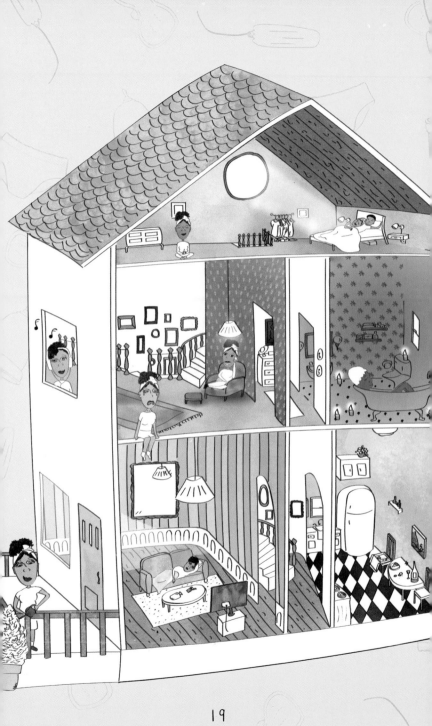

19

YOUR PERIOD HOROSCOPE

Ask a friend to fill in each blank prompt according to their mood. Then read the whole thing out loud and expect uproarious laughter!

_____
(ZODIAC SIGN)

A new _____ might be added to your period.
     (NOUN)

Don't be _____ about finding a used _____
    (EMOTION)   (PERIOD PRODUCT)

in an unusual place (could even be in a _____). It's
                                  (LOCATION)

meant as inspiration! A long-term goal of bleeding

during _____ could finally be _____. As
   (EVENT)   (VERB ENDING IN -ED)

could that long-awaited vacation with a _____
                              (ADJECTIVE)

partner. They'll bring all the _____.
              (PERIOD PRODUCT, PLURAL)

All you need to bring is a love of _____!
                      (ACTIVITY)

When I was just nine years of age,

I was told that my life turned a page.

In the bathroom to pee,

bright red stained my blue jeans,

and now every four weeks I do rage.

—MARTINA PAPINCHAK

PERIOD WORD FIND

```
E N D O M E T R I O S I S J G
Y X P N E U K D J K T W D F J
G D P J N R Q M E N S E S F O
J F O Z S S F E H O O A U Z V
Q N P W T Q G N M E O D J L U
P C C W R J A S P I B L M W L
W E U C U H L T T A M P O N A
T R B R A M P R B B L U X U T
R C J A T P S U A A Y U Y B I
K B X H I R N A H M Q T Q L O
E Y N X O J N L N Y G E Y O N
X A Z A N P T C M U H R E O G
Q C R A M P S U H W N U X D T
C E P P B M Q P P U R S N Y R
```

UTERUS	MENSTRUAL CUP	MENSES
TAMPON	MENSTRUATION	CRAMPS
BLOODY	ENDOMETRIOSIS	OVULATION

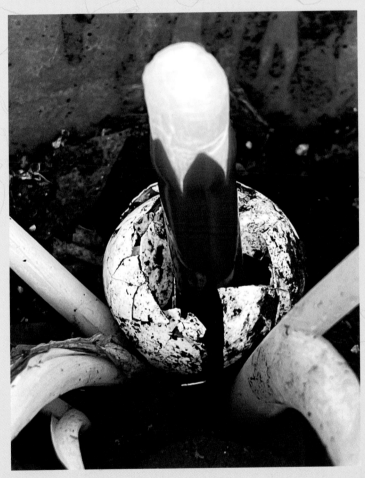

Photo by Neno

"R & D"

By Carissa Kosta

SCENE ONE.
DR. BARBARA BROWNE's lab at SnugPlug headquarters, 1989.

It's adorned with late-eighties-era items: a rotary phone, boombox, etc. In front of her is a set of beakers, different-colored liquids, and tampons along with measuring devices like a small scale and precision ruler. She's in the middle of performing some sort of test.

(BARBARA DIALS)

BARBARA:

Hi, is this the FDA? Great, this is Dr. Browne calling from SnugPlug Research and Development. Ha, yes, the "brains behind the bleed" indeed! I'm looking to speak with someone about a fax I just received stating that the FDA is requiring we place some sort of a chart on the back of tampon boxes to "help" women figure out what size tampon they need. Whose idea was this? Yours! Hm. Mind if I ask a few follow-up questions? Great!

The proposed standardized system includes "'junior,' 'regular,' 'super,' and 'super-plus' absorbency, on a scale from six to fifteen grams." First question: how are women supposed to weigh their flow? Uh huh. Are you suggesting then that we provide an Erlenmeyer flask in every box so she can take a week off of her life and walk around with an inserted flask dangling from her vagina to get an accurate reading? Oh, okay, well...what do you propose?...Hello? Ah, thought I lost you. We can come back to that. Second follow-up question: why, pray tell, is the measurement in the metric system? Here in the US, the only thing we talk about in grams is marijuana. Are you assuming all women who menstruate are potheads?

Also, have there been a considerable number of complaints from women about having a hard time knowing what size tampon they need? Most of the women I know, including myself, have a pretty easy and reliable system: if I used one that wasn't big enough, I stain my undies, and if I used one that was too big, it feels like I'm pulling out a giant saltine.

(BEAT)

Haha, yes, I *have* made mini saltine pizzas! An old boyfriend and I used to make them together all the time. Yes, sliced-up string cheese is the key…. Wait… hold on…is this Stan?? Stan! I knew I recognized your voice. It's me, Barbara! What a riot! Well…you're at the FDA now, congratulations! Odd that *you* of all people are in charge of tampon regulation! When *we* were together, you were grossed out whenever I had my period.

You told me you "can't do the deed while I bleed" because you have a "weak nose."

(BEAT)

Yes, you did. Yes, you absolutely did. You know what? I'm not doing this again. Congratulations on the dumbest idea for a tampon box ever. No, of course I don't want women to get TSS. But, uh oh…you know what? I'm getting 1.4 mL of TSS right now— Toxic Stan Syndrome! Goodbye, Stan!

(SHE HANGS UP)

Barbara downs a sleeve of saltines and the crumbles tumble from her mouth.

FADE TO BLACK.

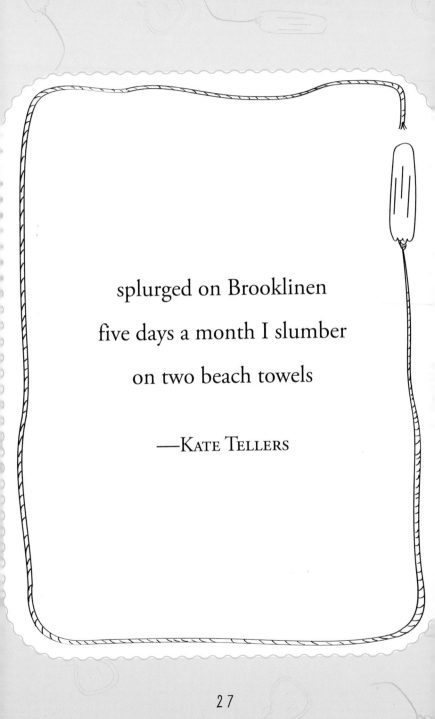

splurged on Brooklinen

five days a month I slumber

on two beach towels

—KATE TELLERS

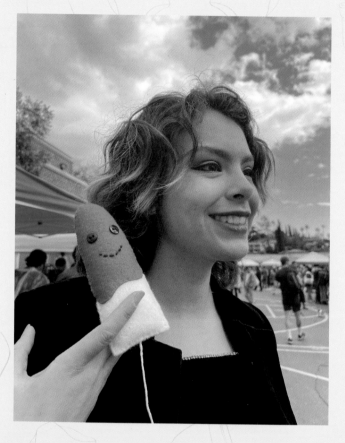

Art by Shelley Friedman (Model: Hannah Sterling)

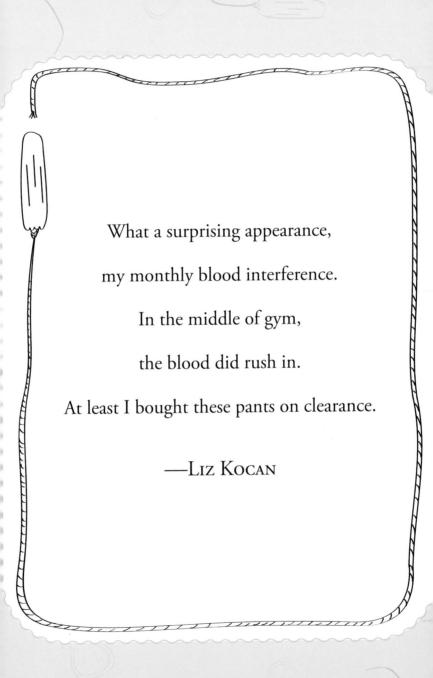

What a surprising appearance,

my monthly blood interference.

In the middle of gym,

the blood did rush in.

At least I bought these pants on clearance.

—Liz Kocan

Representative Sean Patrick Maloney included tampons in his office supply list, you know, for visiting constituents who menstruate. The House's Office of Finance deemed them an "impermissible puchase." So Rep. Maloney wrote out a personal check to cover the $37 and keep those tampons available.

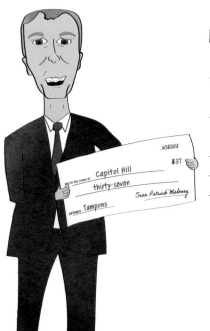

Ways You Too Can Be An Ally:

- Throw a box of tampons in your trunk.
- Don't say "ew" when someone says the word period; just listen.
- Bake cookies.
- Hug someone while they cry it out.
- Suggest a heating pad and your cookies.

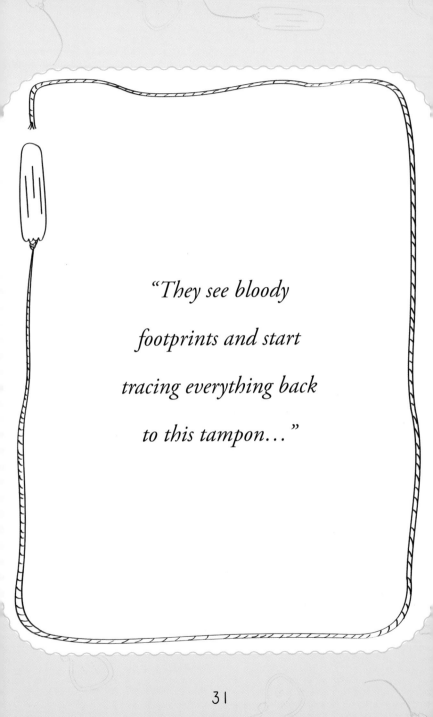

"They see bloody footprints and start tracing everything back to this tampon…"

"THEY SEE BLOODY FOOTPRINTS"

By Lorraine DeGraffenreidt

I got my period for the first time at age twelve on what just happens to be my mother's birthday. She thinks it's awesome, and in general, she finds these kinds of calendar coincidences cute and meaningful. I am indifferent to such coincidences, but even so, I can't help noticing how similarly my mother and I have always treated our periods respectively. We are both pretty neglectful, especially when it comes to tampons. I probably picked this up from her, but if I'm having a busy day, I will wear my tampon for way longer than is recommended by the tampon box instructions. Doctors these days say four to eight hours is the longest you should go without changing your tampon and even at eight hours…you're pushing it. For me, however, eight hours is on the shorter side. I will leave my tampon in for an entire day if I feel like it. I will leave my tampon in overnight and then not change it until the following night's next morning. I. Don't. Care. If toxic shock is still a real threat, it hasn't caught up to me yet.

I remember one particularly busy day for me. It's my senior year in high school. I have a lot going on with schoolwork, my social life, and extracurricular activities. All of my college applications are in, but I'm still the president of a few clubs at school and on the varsity basketball team. It's a game day for my team, by the way, which is a big deal. On game days, the whole team wears their basketball uniforms to school so the student body can be reminded to come out and support. I love this tradition because it means I'm already dressed for my game and don't have to schedule in time to step away and get changed.

Unfortunately, I get my period in the morning while I'm at school. I check to make sure I didn't bleed through my basketball shorts, and luckily, I did not. Since I wasn't expecting to get my period today, I didn't think to bring any tampons to school with me from home, so I go to the nurse's office and grab a free tampon. They only have the cheap, flimsy ones that come with the cardboard applicator. For a busy girl with a medium-to-heavy flow, these tampons are a precarious setup for day-one-of-my-period coverage.

I put my faith in this tampon regardless, and I wear her all day.

After school, my basketball team loads onto the bus and we travel to our game across town. At this point, I have been wearing the free tampon from the nurse's office for many hours—certainly more hours than is recommended on the tampon box. Another detail: I am not wearing spandex. It's just me, the tampon, my underwear, and some swishy, swishy basketball shorts. We are out here, living dangerously today. If you think I took a second at any point before my game to use the restroom and swap out the old tampon for a new one, you are wrong.

During the basketball game, my whole plan of neglecting my tampon is going just fine until I dive onto the ground to fight an opponent for the basketball. Adrenaline flows through my veins while I and another girl are on the ground, both grabbing tightly to the basketball. We are fighting to win what is called a "jump ball." The referees blow their whistles to stop the play and to change possession. This is what happens after a jump ball. As usual, both teams dust themselves off and reset once the possession is changed. We all jog to the opposite end of the court and wait for the referees to blow their whistles indicating that the game may resume. But the game does not resume. We all stand there confused, watching the referees pace around the court where the jump ball struggle just occurred. They appear to be doing forensic detective work once they see bloody footprints and start tracing everything back to this tampon. They're two middle-aged men, quietly conferring with one another, trying to decide what to do about that wet, bloody wad of *something* that is delaying this girls' high school basketball game.

I'm in shock and disbelief when the referees call an emergency timeout and clear the players from the court, sending us to our benches. As I jog over to huddle up with my team by our bench, I'm thinking, "No.... No, no, no, no. *That* could *NOT* be mine!!!!" Then, in the huddle, I'm trying to focus on the game or on anything my coach is saying to us. He's saying things like, "We can't be distracted by whatever is going on over there! Let's focus on what we worked on in practice! We have to be thinking about our plays!" I, of course, cannot think about our plays. I'm watching an athletic trainer lady run onto the court with medical gloves, a few sheets of cotton gauze, and a plastic bag to scoop up the mess. I'm overhearing a couple of teenage boys who are sitting at the score table, operating the score clock. One guy goes, "Dude. You know what that thing is, right?" The other one goes, "DUDE! No way! Do not tell me that's what I think it is!!!" Elsewhere, I'm seeing a woman sitting in the bleachers next to two little boys. They're tugging at her clothes, begging her to explain what's going on like, "Mom! Mom! There's blood on the floor! Explain this to us! What is that blood?!" In a discreet, curt tone she says, "Don't worry, boys. We'll talk about it in the car."

As is expected, the game resumes, and no one specific person gets called out for the rogue tampon mess. I continue playing, to finish the game strong, as if nothing is wrong. Because, like, you know what? Why should anything be wrong?! There's still hope, right?! Maybe that loose tampon wasn't actually mine! It's still possible. I mean, after everything went down, I had my buddy check me out and she saw no evidence of any blood anywhere on me. Not on my swishy, swishy basketball shorts. Not on my legs. Not even on the bottoms of my shoes! There was nothing.

But also…as is expected…when I finally do get a minute to check things out in the bathroom…I find even more nothing. The free tampon from the nurse's office has completely disappeared. So, I guess that totally was my tampon on the court. For sure. But how? HOW?! How is this even possible?! I still do not know. My tampon wriggled free. She said, "HELLO! And GOODBYE! I am a bloody tampon and I will *not* be neglected!!" All of this being said, I no longer trust tampons. I mean, I do still wear them…I just don't trust them. Every time I'm wearing one, I'm wondering if it's really still in there. I'm never sure.

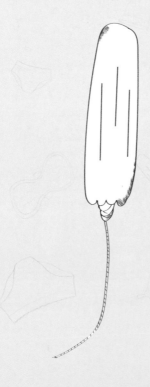

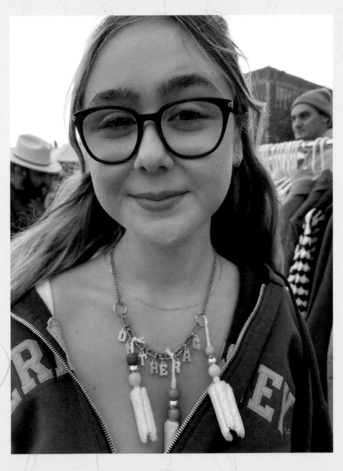

Art by Shelley Friedman (Model: Mazzy Miziker)

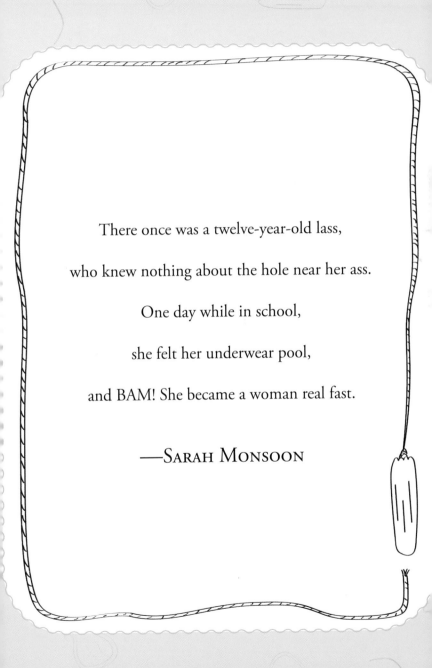

There once was a twelve-year-old lass,

who knew nothing about the hole near her ass.

One day while in school,

she felt her underwear pool,

and BAM! She became a woman real fast.

—Sarah Monsoon

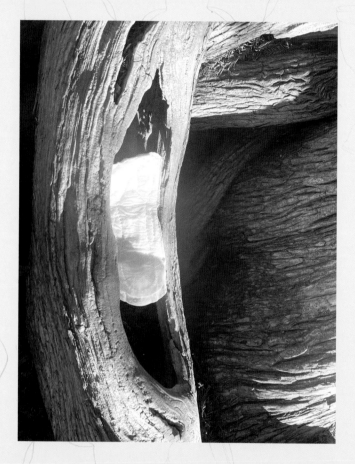

Photo by Neno

PERIOD PLAYLISTS

When you have your period, sometimes you just
want to put on some music and laugh or cry
or cry while laughing.

Here are some jams that will help you do just that!

EMPOWHER!!!!

I Love It - Icona Pop (feat. Charli XCX)

I AM - Baby Tate (feat. Flo Milli)

Truth Hurts - Lizzo

No - Meghan Trainor

Don't Take It Personal - Monica

Roar - Katy Perry

IDGAF - Dua Lipa

Like a Girl - Lizzo

Fire Woman - The Cult

I'll Show You Crazy - JOEY DJIA

Another One Bites the Dust - Queen

You Can't Hurry Love - The Supremes

Let it Bleed - The Rolling Stones

Girl on Fire - Alicia Keys

Love Myself - Hailee Steinfeld

Respect - Aretha Franklin

Run the World - Beyoncé

I Wanna Dance with Somebody - Whitney Houston

Redneck Woman - Gretchen Wilson

My Humps - Black Eyed Peas

Glamorous - Fergie

Fight Song - Rachel Platten

Brave - Sara Bareilles

That's Alright - Laura Mvula

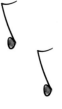

Get Your Cry On

Let Her Go - Passenger
Sunday Bloody Sunday - U2
I'm a Woman - Koko Taylor
Let it Go - James Bay
Just Give Me a Reason - Pink
On My Own - Les Misérables
Big Girls Don't Cry - Fergie
Life Ain't Always Beautiful - Gary Allan
Piece by Piece - Kelly Clarkson*
Too Late to Turn Back Now - Cornelius Brothers and Sister Rose
Say Something - A Great Big World and Christina Aguilera
Teenage Dream - T. Rex
There Goes My Baby - The Drifters
Landslide - Fleetwood Mac
Boyish - Japanese Breakfast
More Than a Woman - The Bee Gees
Patience - Tame Impala
Venus as a Boy - Björk
All Things Must Pass - George Harrison
I'm Just Snacking - Gus Dapperton

* bonus points for the American Idol version where she couldn't get through it without crying

43

SWEET EMOTIONS

You will feel all of the emotions before, during, and after your period. FUN!

They are all valid.

You are valid.

These emotions include
(but are not limited to)...

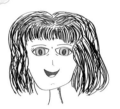

HAPPY

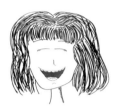

THRILLED

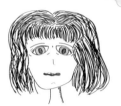

ANXIOUS

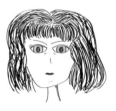

ANGRY

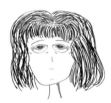

EXHAUSTED

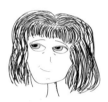

THOUGHTFUL

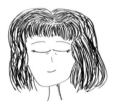

CALM

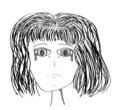

OVERWHELMED

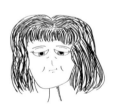

SICK

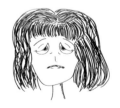

DEFEATED

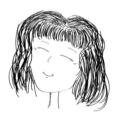

EMPOWERED

SHY

45

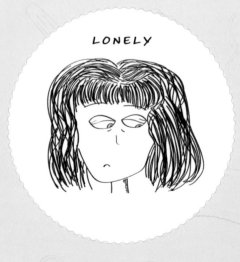

LONELY

"HER NAME WAS ROXY"

By Steph Garcia

Roxy was a force. I loved waking up every morning to her warm body in my bed. Watching her slumbering face was my comfort. She could be incredibly stubborn, but I knew it was because she was astoundingly intelligent.

So, I could look past her stubbornness. It was almost endearing honestly. But there was one thing she did that always enraged me.

She ripped up my dirty pads. Just tore them up. With her teeth.

My wonderful pup Roxy loved getting into the garbage whenever it was that time of the month. She was like a kid in a candy store…if candy was period blood encased in pads and the only way to get it out was by leaving bits throughout my house.

I read on the internet a few theories about the dog thinking of me as the "alpha" and being attracted to

47

the scent or wanting to rip up the scent so as not to attract predators. I don't know. It's the internet.

What I do know is that it was embarrassing. Like, the last thing you want as a young teen is for someone to come over and find a shredded, bloody mound on your welcome mat. Because that blonde beauty Roxy loved to coat our hallways, and sometimes our beds, with her debris.

Fortunately, Roxy had a lot of great traits. She was fantastic at doing tricks! When she wanted to do them. She was stubborn, remember?

Roxy definitely made me precious as to where I placed my used menstruation products when I got my first dog as an adult. But, aside from also being a four-letter-starting-with-R-named-wonder, my next dog, Ruby, was nothing like Roxy. Ruby wouldn't dare touch the pizza box we left on our coffee table, even if no human was home, much less my trashed bloody products.

My teenage self was very jealous. No destruction, plus way less people to be embarrassed by it! Or maybe I just became more comfortable with the whole idea of a period. Maybe it was a combination. I don't know. It's the internet.

Wait, this isn't the internet. This is a book. You get it.

I love my dogs.

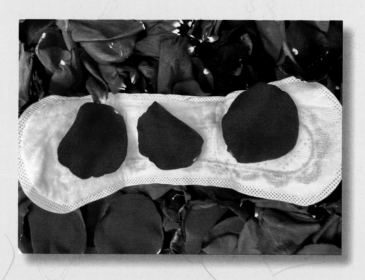

Photo by Neno

"SCHOOL BATHROOMS AS A TRANS MAN"

By Levi Yates

I am an eighth grader. Which means my school is full of awkward teenagers who don't like to admit that they're as awkward as they are. And with that, there are only a few "out" trans people. Being transgender in middle school is very odd. Especially when you have to go to the bathroom.

In my case, I look too masculine to use the girls' bathroom. But too feminine to use the boys' bathroom. But not androgynous enough to alternate. I pass as much as I can for being fourteen and overweight. But still, it's not enough for cis people at my school. My voice isn't always as low as I want it to be, and I don't wear my binder every day. The masks definitely help, but as soon as I take mine off, it goes downhill.

How do you solve a problem like that? I just stopped using the bathrooms at school.

Oftentimes when I used the school bathrooms, the girls in there would give me looks of confusion and sometimes disgust. I would always just walk into a stall and wait for people to leave. Or for someone else to flush. I am someone who hated public bathrooms even before I realized I was trans. I hate the concept of sitting on the same toilet as someone five minutes after they leave.

I overheard someone once saying to their friend, "Oh my gosh did you see that—" and then they walked out, so I actually have no idea if they misgendered me or not. I stayed in that bathroom until no one else was in there. Which was a pretty long time because it was right before my lunch period.

Speaking of periods, they add another layer of awkwardness for trans middle schoolers. If you go into the girls' bathroom, you get weird looks. If you go into the boys' bathroom, there are no trash cans in the stalls. And can you imagine the anxiety you would feel as you rip the pad off, while other cis boys are in the room wondering what that noise is? It's almost worse than doing that in the girls' bathroom.

Another good reason to avoid school bathrooms, if you ask me.

If you're a transgender middle schooler like me and you also hate public bathrooms, I have a tip for dealing with your period at school.

My tip for trans guys who aren't on testosterone and are in school currently is this: POCKETS. Big, deep pockets. You need a bag with big pockets. And you need pants or a hoodie with big pockets. Especially if you use pads. If you use tampons, this should still work. I have a canvas messenger bag, and since I don't use the school bathrooms, I don't carry pads every day. But if my flow is very heavy that day, I will slide one or two pads into wherever I can. As a bookmark, in my notebooks, whatever. But when I had a backpack, I had an entire pocket devoted to this kind of thing. The pocket had two or three pads, and then, if I had come back from my dad's house (my parents are divorced), there might be some spare underwear that I forgot to unpack. Then when you know you have to go to the bathroom to change your pad, use a little trickery. Start by grabbing something from your bag like a notebook and then put it back and make it seem like you forgot something. That's when you grab the thing you really need—the pad. Put it in your pocket immediately and go.

If you're a trans man who is as awkward as I am in school bathrooms, then I really hope this helped. Even if it inspired a way to be secretive about period supplies, I'll be glad.

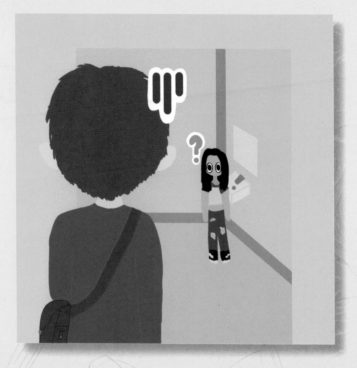

Illustration by Levi Yates

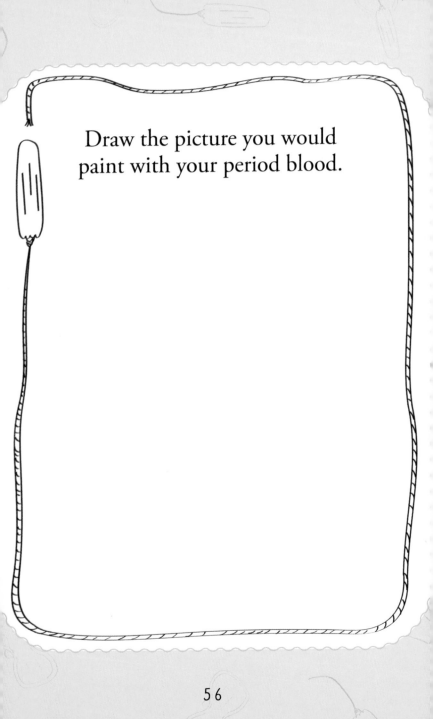

Draw the picture you would
paint with your period blood.

"FLOW HIT ME"
By Lori Elberg

When I was two, I entered my first Jewish pre-school. When I was five, I started Hebrew school. My parents schooled me on the Jewishness of every Hollywood extra and off-off-Catskill comedian. My upbringing included Jewish traditions, both cultural and religious. When I discovered the gap in my Jewish education, it felt like a slap in the face.

I was twelve years old—a shy, awkward kid. My mother, Flo, had me when she was in her forties, so my references were dated. I could name more songs by Frank Sinatra than the New Kids on the Block. Maybe if I was less interested in collecting stickers and more interested in obtaining hickeys from brace-faced boys at camp, the girls in my bunk would have prepared me. I was the kid who knew nothing—the last girl to get her period.

I remember that summer before the flow hit me. The girls in the bunk came with trunkloads of pads. Our counselor, a teased-hair, gum-chewing sixteen-year-old from Long Island, had tampons in more sizes than a Russian nesting doll. This poor schmuck named Danielle had a colossal pad with straps that she wore like a holster under her days-of-the-week underwear. I missed the starlight screening of *Grease 2* when I had to escort Danielle to the nurse because she ran out of her medieval pads. She cried as the nurse placed a special order that sadly wouldn't arrive in time to finish her cycle. That summer was educational. I was confident I was ready for menstruation. I was going to get my period that summer! I was wrong.

In September, I entered junior high. I got boobs that appeared overnight. It felt unfair that I skipped that cute little AAA boobies phase and went straight to a large B cup, complete with hips. My mother took me to the Wizard of Bras, a shop where old Jewish women get their brassieres. There, in that dusty back room, I was initiated into the tribe. This tribe consisted of old ladies sucked into girdles, garters, and corsets. My mother told tales of her first trip to a bra shop in Brooklyn. It was a moment she and her mother shared. Flo was beaming with pride.

A woman in her late forties, which seemed ancient at the time, opened the curtain unannounced and stared at my naked torso. The cigarette dangling from her mouth ashed and burned a small hole in my Keds. She lifted my arms, cupped my boobs, and wrapped me in a tape measure. She called me "Hon" and threw boxes around as she talked about my perky bubs. Smokey busted into the dressing room. She pointed out how supportive the ACE-bandage-colored-bras were on my young figure.

Would it have felt more like a rite of passage if Flo simply took me to the mall? I learned that Jew-berty is more about humiliation than transformation, and this was just the beginning…

It's Yom Kippur, and I'm dizzy. The Jewish day of atonement, the only holiday that is more about not eating than eating.

This strange feeling must be because I didn't eat.

My stomach hurts.

Did I just pee myself?

I rush to the bathroom.

I see it—biology!

The period to this humiliating sentence—

I am a woman.

I call to Flo to tell her about my flow.

She rushes into the bathroom.

SLAP!

OW! What the f— just happened?

FLO HIT ME! A slap clear across the face.

I hold both my cheek and my tears.

"Are you mad at me? Did I do something wrong?"

She beams with pride. "Not at all, sweetie, it's a tradition. Mazel tov!"

"WHAT?" I feel violated. What kind of tradition involves slapping your daughter when she is dizzy, bleeding, and hungry?

Did this at least mean I could eat now?

If *Cathy* comics taught me anything, it was that I am at least entitled to ice cream. Is Cathy Jewish? Does menstruation cancel out atonement? What kind of patriarchal BS is this slapping across the face?

The slap was not playful. It was a slap like you see in old movies and sitcoms (probably penned by masochistic Jewish writers). The slap a character gives when someone needs to "snap out of it." A slap to replace smelling salts or cold water on the face of someone who fainted.

This slap was a whack.

My mother had never hit me. I was shocked.

What was crazy was that this was a tradition? Why was I so unprepared?

In Hebrew school, we learned about mikvahs—splish splash, it's a Jewish period bath. I had my ten thousand hours in Judaism and never was there a mention of the slap.

After some internet research, I found that the "menstrual slap" is not an officially sanctioned practice in Judaism. I assumed every Jewish girl had the same experience. We never mentioned it again. I was reminded years later during a viewing of the movie *A Walk on the Moon*. In the film, young Alison, played by Anna Paquin, has a similar experience with her bubbe. Finally, confirmation that my mother wasn't just a masochist. It was a tradition! An awful tradition, yes, but probably less damaging than Smokey the bra-bandit. The slap healed, the story remained.

Now in my forties, I have asked my Jewish peers, and I was shocked to find that very few had experienced the slap. Was it because my mom was older? Did the women's movement kill the menstrual slap? What about those girls in my bunk? Is it an East Coast thing? An Ashkenazi practice?

I am now the mother of a daughter. She is several years away from becoming a woman. Will I slap her in the face? No. I will tell her about the day her grandma Flo hit me, kiss her on the cheeks, and say, "Mazel tov!"

I will tell her that while we learn about our history and our culture, not every tradition needs to be observed. I will tell her about the years of pain and discomfort that come with menstruation. She will not feel the pain or confusion from a slap across the face. I'm confident she will find other humiliating events in her upbringing to talk about thirty years later.

PERIOD PREPAREDNESS

GAH!! You've literally started your period.

Again.

It's the cycle of life, a beautiful thing, and blah, blah, blah.

Now it's time to be prepared.

Here are some helpful handy-dandy survival pack ideas/suggestions/necessities to thrive in the world while bleeding.

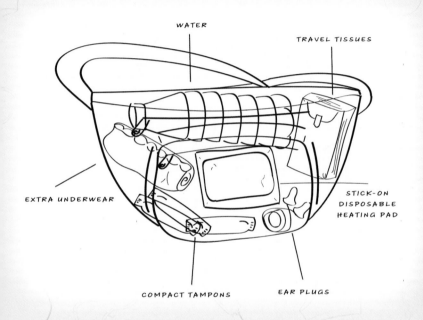

WATER

TRAVEL TISSUES

EXTRA UNDERWEAR

STICK-ON
DISPOSABLE
HEATING PAD

COMPACT TAMPONS

EAR PLUGS

The Beloved Fanny Pack: Strap this puppy across your midsection, or swing it across your chest while hiking, powering through a busy intersection, on the way to your midterms, or in a busy airport terminal prepping to fly first class —like the boss you are! Compact, light, and ready for action!

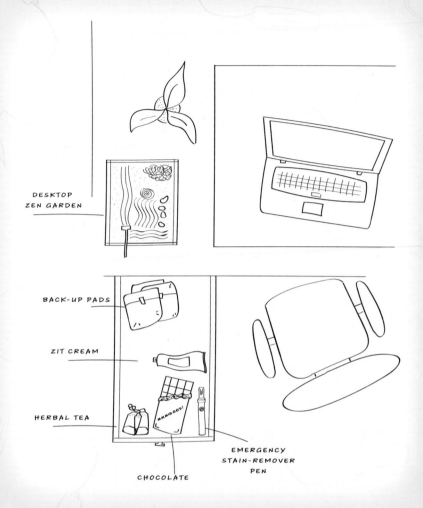

DESKTOP
ZEN GARDEN

BACK-UP PADS

ZIT CREAM

HERBAL TEA

CHOCOLATE

EMERGENCY
STAIN-REMOVER
PEN

Make It Work for You at Work: Love/hate or hate/love your job—let your desk be an oasis of escape. Stock up with goodies to create ease and comfort. Don't forget the backup pads! Who KNOWS how long Darryl will make you stay late in order to get that promotion you already deserve!

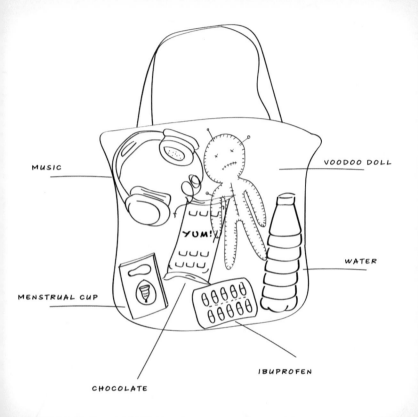

MUSIC

VOODOO DOLL

YUM!

WATER

MENSTRUAL CUP

IBUPROFEN

CHOCOLATE

Tote's Tote: This thing carries it all. Durable, trustworthy, functional, a little worse-for-wear, and full of hidden goodies—just like you! Carry this through life, armed against the masses. You, your bag, and some black magic from the aisles of Trader Joe's.

IT'S TIME FOR...PERIOD JOKES!

With Kristine Kimmel & Jessie Gaskell

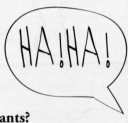

What's the safest time to wear white pants?

At your funeral.

How can you tell if your friend is wearing a menstrual cup?

Don't worry, she'll tell you.

Knock knock.

Who's there?

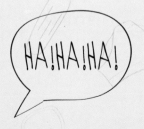

Go check your underwear.

Damnit.

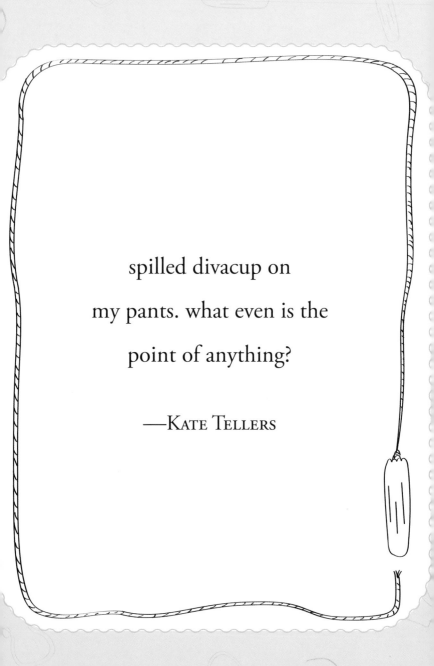

spilled divacup on

my pants. what even is the

point of anything?

—KATE TELLERS

"A LESSON ON PUBERTY"

By Kay Kaanapu

It was a temperate summer Sunday when my mother and aunt were chatting in the kitchen. I was a ten-year-old bookworm about to start the sixth grade, so I read quietly at the kids' table. I was engrossed in the newest saga of the Sleepover Friends, a preteen novel series that was basically a knock-off of The Baby-Sitters Club. As the daughter of two teachers, my middle-class upbringing was populated by the generic versions of mainstream brand names.

Books usually whisked me so far away from normal life, but for some reason, a word my aunt uttered broke through my focus. I looked up and asked, "Mom, what does 'puberty' mean?" The eyes of my mother and aunt widened with shock. My aunt whispered, "You still haven't told her?" My mother responded by sending me to my room. Minutes later she appeared with my sister, who was a year younger than me. My mother turned on the TV, put a tape into the VCR, set a timer for ninety minutes, and said, "Don't come out until this timer goes off and if you have any questions, ask your dad." Then she pressed play and left.

I had no idea what hellfire I had wrought. The tape was an educational, animated video about human reproduction and described the changes to boys' and girls' growing bodies when they hit puberty. It only lasted an hour. So, once the video ended, my sister and I were left with a solid thirty minutes to awkwardly sit in silence, avoiding eye contact and feeling icky about our bodies. Tons of questions swirled in my brain, but when the timer finally rang, there was no way my sister and I were going to my dad for answers. We didn't want to discuss our bodies through football and weightlifting metaphors. It wouldn't be until years later, after both my sisters and I had already progressed through puberty, that we'd speak to our mother about this incident. But on that day, we didn't talk about it. I just went back to my book.

A couple months into sixth grade, the teachers announced a special lesson. It involved separating the boys and girls into different rooms, pulling out the TV and VCR units, and showing us a video. To my amused surprise, it was the same tape my mother played for me and my sister. I felt like I had received an early screening of a life-changing blockbuster because I knew the big twist ending. After they reintegrated the classrooms, everyone was steaming with awkward ick and suspiciously eyeing each other's bodies. Except me. Because I had already seen the video and was acquainted with its knowledge.

At lunch, a boy from my class noticed I wasn't as shook as the rest of them. While he "ew"-ed over every detail from the video, I just offered knowing giggles. He demanded, "How come you're not weirded out?" I proudly stated, "I already saw it." However, he heard, "I already got it." He proceeded to scream, "You already got it? You already got your period? Hey! Kay already got her period." He repeated this over and over while cackling at the top of his lungs. "No. I said I already saw it. I already saw it." But the damage was done. I became the girl that already got her period, even though I truly hadn't.

To battle the bullying, I found strength in wearing my favorite piece of clothing—my yellow shorts. I loved these yellow shorts because when I wore them, I felt like the Yellow Power Ranger. I was a huge *Power Rangers* fan. We're talking about the OG 90s version that aired on US TV. And I was obsessed with the

Yellow Ranger. She was an Asian girl named Trini and always dressed in yellow. Sure, this element of the show was a bit racist especially since the Black Ranger was also a Black guy who always dressed in black. But Trini was an Asian, female superhero on television. She made me feel seen, so I loved her and the show. My yellow shorts made me feel strong and kick-ass just like the Yellow Ranger, especially when I was teased for having a nonexistent period.

Then on a slightly chilly winter day, I wore my shorts and played handball at recess. I could not lose. I was on a run and hitting everyone out. I even cycled through the line of incoming players at least twice. Suddenly, I had this overwhelming sensation to go to the bathroom. After negotiating a deal to not lose my winning streak and verifying I could jump back into the game upon my return, I ran to the bathroom. That's where I first noticed a reddish-brown streak near the front of my underwear. But I was too focused on the handball and the power of the shorts surging through me, so I ignored it. I was the Yellow Ranger. Nothing would stop me.

But when I got home from school, the stain was even bigger and had leaked onto my shorts. It still didn't occur to me that it was my period. Instead, I assumed that I hadn't wiped my butt sufficiently after a poop. I debated whether or not to mention it to my mother. And I probably wouldn't have if the stain hadn't affected my shorts. I loved those shorts so much that it was worth asking my mother if she could work her magic and repair them to their full yellow color. So, unlike the day when I first learned about puberty, I talked to my mother. She looked at them, casually shook her head, and said, "No, you'll have to get new shorts. That's a period stain." I was devastated. Not about getting my period, but about losing my beloved shorts. I never found another pair with that special alchemy of fabric and color that made me feel both comfortable and strong. I could no longer harness the power of the Yellow Ranger.

My mother eventually became comfortable discussing periods with me and my sisters. The subject was less taboo once our household had to deal with the brutal reality of having four menstruating women synced under the same roof. Once a month, we'd suddenly become snippy and short with each other, exchanging eyerolls and cutting comments. Only then did our conversation turn to buying pads and tampons and medication for our cramps.

I don't plan on having children, so I doubt I'll experience teaching my daughter about puberty and her period. But if I ever impart knowledge about these touchy subjects to a young girl, I hope she'd feel free to ask questions. I'd try to give her information without judgement and help her view her body through a scientific lens, detached from the moral weight that society heaps upon women. So many living creatures in nature reproduce, but humanity is one of the few species that can directly communicate about reproduction. We should thrive in this privilege and be comfortable talking to each other. Especially when you're a mother and your daughter just asked, "What does 'puberty' mean?"

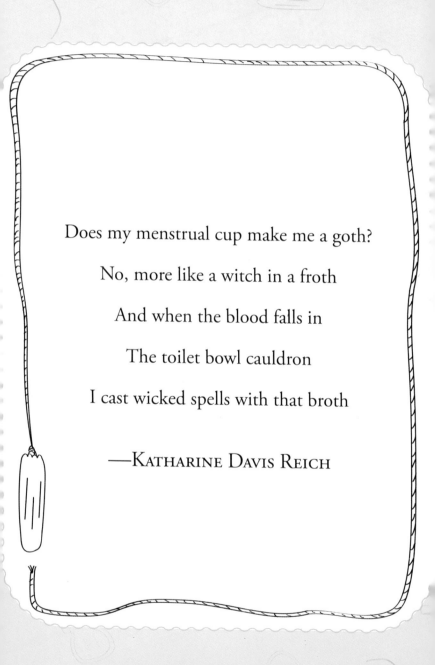

Does my menstrual cup make me a goth?

No, more like a witch in a froth

And when the blood falls in

The toilet bowl cauldron

I cast wicked spells with that broth

—Katharine Davis Reich

MONTH

S	M	T	W	Th	F	S
		1	2	3	4	5
6	7	8	9	10	11	12
13	14	15	16	17	18	19
20	21	22	23	24	25	26
27	28	29	30			

'TWAS THE NIGHT BEFORE

Ask a friend to fill in each blank prompt according to their mood. Then read the whole thing out loud and expect uproarious laughter!

'Twas the night before _____when all I
(SPECIAL OCCASION)

could _____
(VERB)

was my period bleeding right through my _____.
(NOUN)

The _____ were stocked in the bathroom with
(PERIOD PRODUCT, PLURAL)

_____.
(EMOTION)

And I hoped that my bleeding soon would be _____.
(VERB WITH ING)

I grabbed one to nestle, and got snug in my _____
(NOUN)

While visions of _____ danced in my _____.
        (NOUN)   (BODY PART)

My momma used _____ and now I use _____.
            (PERIOD PRODUCT)   (PERIOD PRODUCT)

But with all this bleeding, I would even use _____.
                                        (NOUN, PLURAL)

Then out in the _____ there arose such a clatter!
              (LOCATION)

My partner brought _____ to cover the splatter!
                (NOUN, PLURAL)

Away from the toilet, I flew like a _____.
                                (NOUN)

For tomorrow was saved and tonight was a _____.
                                    (NOUN)

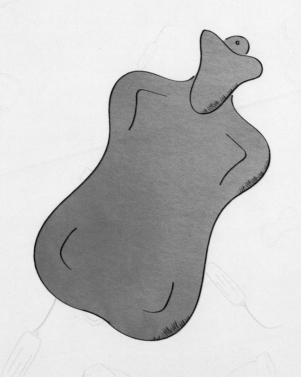

IT'S TIME AGAIN FOR...
PERIOD JOKES!

With Kristine Kimmel & Jessie Gaskell

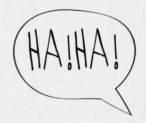

What's the one thing every menstrual cup wearer needs?

A backup plan.

What's the difference between an Amazon package and my period?

I know how to track an Amazon package.

What's black and brown and red all over?

Every single crotch of my underwear.

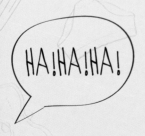

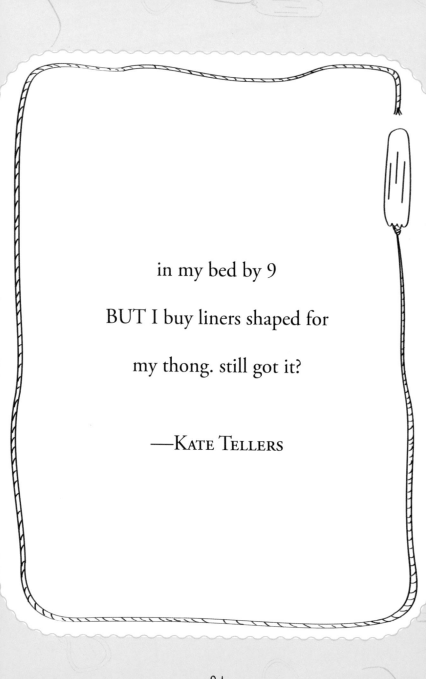

in my bed by 9

BUT I buy liners shaped for

my thong. still got it?

—KATE TELLERS

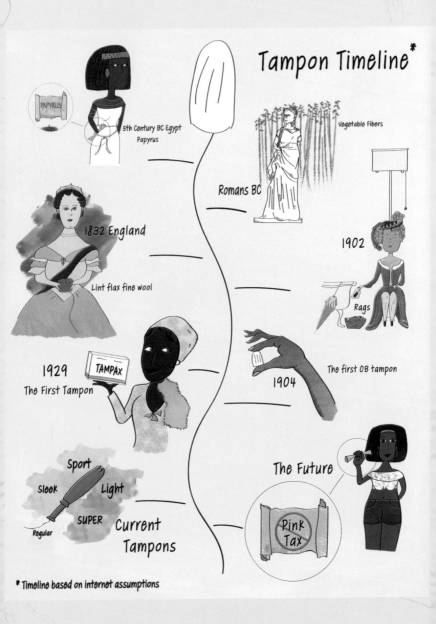

Tampon Timeline*

5th Century BC Egypt
Papyrus
PAPYRUS

Romans BC
Vegetable Fibers

1832 England
Lint flax fine wool

1902
Rags

1929
The First Tampon
TAMPAX

1904
The first OB tampon

Sport
Sleek
Light
Regular
SUPER
Current
Tampons

The Future
Pink
Tax

* Timeline based on internet assumptions

"THE KOTEX BELT"

By Jessica Shein

Like most girls of a certain age, I became obsessed with getting my period, the first in what I thought were a series of steps to becoming a bona fide adult. But I was eighty-nine pounds, flat-chested, with nary a hair on my pubis. In other words, I wasn't destined to be the first, third, or twentieth girl in my class to get my period. But I was undeterred by nature, and instead attempted to coax out my first menstrual cycle by wearing pads every day, as if my ovaries could sense the super absorbent cotton I'd affixed to my underpants and think, "It's go time." When that didn't work, I found tampons, which were not even yet discussed amongst my peers. Figuring the instructions for insertion were grossly incorrect, I instead laid the cotton swab horizontally into the lips of my vulva, its string hanging like some sort of white flag for my childhood.

When my period finally did arrive (while visiting my dad, hours before he threw a huge party for my grandmother's birthday, but that's a whole other embarrassing fiasco), I was elated and eager for guidance from my mother, who at that point I still thought knew all. Tucked under the blankets in my bed, a heating pad pressing against my first brush with cramps, she presented me with what she referred to as a "Kotex belt." Made up of white elastic that fit around my waist, along with two plastic clips that conveniently attached to each end of the pad, my mom explained that the device was once popular and useful. I needn't worry about leakage when this all-powerful strap kept my "napkin" in place. And she was right. Through three middle-of-the-night changes, those pads stayed put. Confidently, the next morning, I slipped the belt on beneath my underwear and went to school.

By 8 a.m., I'd gathered my friends around my locker and announced that I'd gotten my period. There were squeals all around. "I'm wearing the belt now too," I casually added, tugging at my waistband for emphasis.

And then there was a silence that was so loud it felt like a foghorn was blaring in my ear. My face turned as red as the very blood that was collecting in my super-plus-ultra-absorbing-maxi-with-wings. Not one of these girls had heard about this magical period belt; the only belts they wore were chunky and from the Gap or Benetton. I rushed to class, shamed and cursing my mom. At home that night I stuffed the belt into the farthest reaches of my underwear drawer and vowed never to take advice from her again, which I've largely stuck to in the twenty-five years since.

Recently, I rediscovered the elastic artifact while cleaning up my old bedroom. I charged into my mom's room and tossed the belt onto her bed.

"Remember that?" I asked accusingly, like I was confronting a murder suspect with a new piece of evidence.

My mom leaned in and inspected it as if it were some sort of prehistoric fossil. "Wasn't it helpful?" she asked earnestly, completely unaware of how that one item had decimated her credibility in my mind's eye for years.

"It was, yeah, I guess." In an instant I relived the shame from my friends while feeling sad for my mom, who had just wanted to help. Saying nothing more, I grabbed the belt and put it back in the dresser in my childhood room, where it sits today alongside woven bracelets from friends, secret notes passed around in algebra class, and even a few of the old pamphlets from my middle school nurse, explaining what my ovaries and uterus do.

I've thrown out a lot over the years, but I can't seem to toss these items. I think it's because they're a reminder of the relationships we form as we grow up, and how our allegiances change over time. They're also full of stories I'll tell my own daughter one day, pulling out the slim white belt that looks like a torture device and reminiscing about my first period. I won't suggest she wear it, but I'll definitely tell her the right way to use a tampon.

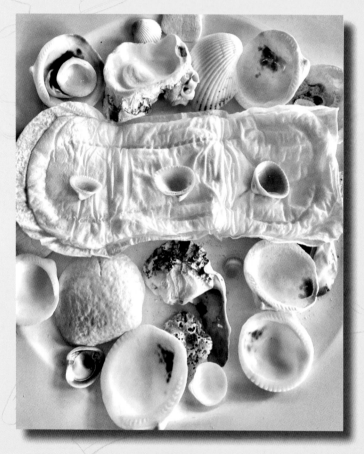

Photo by Neno

"THE MENSTRUAL CUP"

By Emily Churchill

For many years, I've tried to be as environmentally conscious as I can. But the one thing that has eluded me is the menstrual cup. Now, I know that it is better for the environment and my pocketbook, but I just couldn't wrap my brain around it until five months ago. Now, I am a woman who has been through about twenty, plus or minus, years of periods, and I have my rhythm down—or so I thought. But I want to do better for the environment and would love to have less hassle during my periods. Menstrual cup? I've heard good things!

So five months ago I say, "Let's try it! How bad can it be?"

I do my research and find the one I think fits me and helps others. I order two—you know, one to clean while using the other one, right?! And I order the sanitizer, to-go container, and all the bells and whistles. I am getting really excited to use this "menstrual cup"!

They say it's a revolution. I am ready for the revolution!

I get my package in the mail, in time for my upcoming monthly visit! I am ready. I sanitize both cups and get the sanitizer ready on my bathroom counter for when I need to use it. Locked and loaded!

I check my calendar and see that my period should be coming any day now, and having experienced it for many years, it is pretty consistent. Perfect.

A few days later, having forgotten my upcoming excursion for the moment, I look down and realize "IT'S HERE!" I get to use my menstrual cups and do good for the environment and all humankind!

Cool, I am feeling really good about myself and the situation.

So I get the smaller of the two, because I am thinking, this one is probably easier to work with. I think for a moment, "Why were they advertising lube for the cup???!" I'll be fine!

Let's do this!

I read the instructions carefully, multiple times, seeing how it is supposed to work, but not actually knowing how it is going to go down—but I am still optimistic.

I have the cup in my hand and have the instructions right in front of me and think, "We are going in!"

Now, I fold it the way the instructions tell me to, but it keeps coming undone as I am trying to insert it into my vagina. I would say it took me about twenty tries that first time. I am sweating by the end; my shoulder feels like it's going to fall off. Once I finally get the cup in, I feel like I have just run a twenty-six-mile marathon…but it is in! It's in, right??? I can't feel anything—that is good, right??

I read over all the instructions again and, yes, I think I have it in. Whew! Cool!

Wait, is that how it is going to be every time?

Ain't nobody got time for that!

I take a minute and relish the fact that it is in place. And I am not spotting, so that is a sign it is correctly inserted. The language in the instructions makes it sound so easy. I got this!

So then two hours later, I think, "Okay, time to change it! This will be no problem!"

I get the instructions out again, this time for taking it out, and sit down to do this!

I go in, trying to locate the cup. Got it! I feel it, but it is a slip 'n slide down there and I am having a bit of trouble trying to get a hold of it. As I am trying to find it again and again, I read the instructions for getting the cup out. Okay, my fingers keep slipping, and it is NOT as easy as the instructions say. After fifteen minutes of hard-core struggle, I am now panicking and thinking, "I am gonna have to go to the hospital to get this thing out!!!"

I am now sweating, exhausted, and definitely thinking I have dislocated my shoulder in the process, but still no sign of the menstrual cup releasing inside of me.

Twenty-five minutes later, I get a hold of the ribbed part of the cup—this is the goal of getting the cup out of my vagina—and am able to release it and take it out of me.

At that moment, the heavens open up and there is a resounding "AHHHHHHHH!" sound from above.

I empty the contents into the toilet (another thing I am still working through).

And instead of trying my way with the other cup, I opt for a tampon for the time being, because I need to get my bearings about me after that bloody massacre that just took place.

I have gotten better over the last few months and can use my menstrual cup sporadically throughout my period, but every time I think to myself, "I have never been this intimate with my vagina before!" And I do not shy away from my vagina and all my womanhood, but I am still wrapping my brain around the whole concept of the menstrual cup. So I say to you, "Go for it with gusto, but know it will take a lot of faulty tries, a lot of blood (pun intended), sweat, and tears, and you will come out on the other side, helping yourself and the environment! All for Momma Earth. She gets it and loves us for it!"

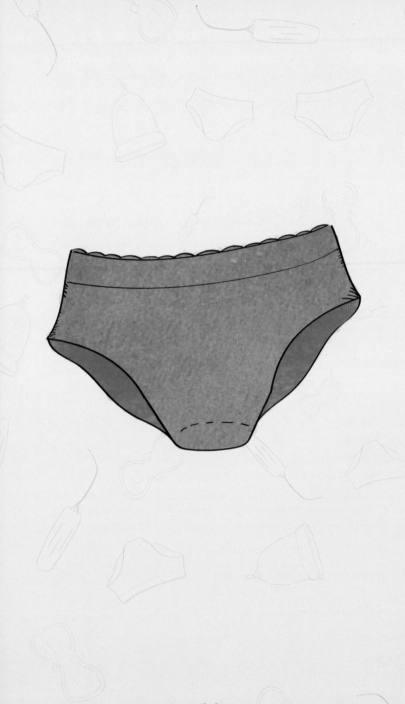

How to: Throw Your Own Period Party

Isn't it fun and not cringeworthy at all to throw your coming of age friend/daughter/niece a super period party celebrating the floodgates opening up and blood spilling in?

Here are things you can do to make your party even more fabulous.

Roll out the red carpet!

Give your period a name! Wait until the end of the party to release it!

Whack a fun tampon-shaped piñata filled with ibuprofen-shaped candy, vagina lapel pins, and diaphragm bracelets.

Fill menstrual cups with fruity punch.

Play pin the maxi pad on the undies.

Yummy! Serve red velvet cake tastefully proclaiming, "You're finally bleeding!" in red letters.

Ps - dont forget to invite their crush!

Party on, period people!

*** But seriously, treat yourself and your body too! You're bleeding. It can hurt and suck and be scary. Do something nice! Nails, a book, and an extra long nap. And if you want to throw a party – do it! See tips above.

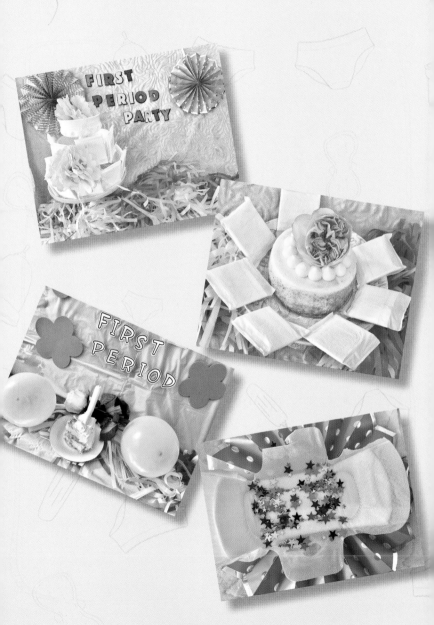

Photos by Neno

95

In 2015, Kiran Gandhi realized she was going to be on her period when she was meant to run for the 26.2 miles of the London Marathon. Gandhi usually avoided running on her period because of the pain, but the day of the marathon coincided with the first day of her period. So instead of forgoing the marathon, she decided to forgo any menstruation product and bleed away!

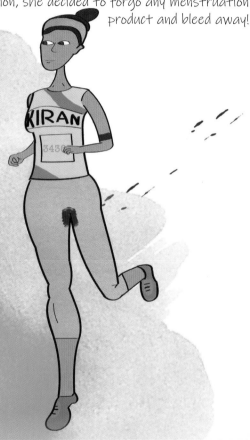

TRUE OR FALSE

1. You can get pregnant during your period.
2. You shouldn't swim during your period.
3. Your period should last exactly one week, once a month.
4. PMS is made-up.
5. You can donate period blood.
6. You lose one pint of blood during your period.
7. Chocolate is good for your period.
8. Periods are something to be ashamed of.
9. Toxic shock syndrome isn't real.

1. True 2. False 3. Depends on the person 4. Super false 5. True 6. False. 2–3 tablespoons is "typical." Consult your doctor if you are losing more. 7. True. Thank you, magnesium. 8. Super false 9. False

"BRUNCH. PERIOD."

By Susie Mendoza

There are many discreet ways to celebrate your daughter's transition into womanhood. Here are a few: (1) buy a sparkly purse to show her impulse purchase are the only real antidote for cramps; (2) tell her a hilarious tale about forgetting tampons at your college graduation as you privately hand her pads; or (3) give her a private hug, whispering, "Congratulations," in a non-creepy way—NOT like that guy in that song, "Lady in Red."

As I stared at the bright red plate in front of me on the momentous day of my first period, I realized with horror that my mother had not chosen any of these options.

Here are some ways to NOT celebrate your daughter's first period: (1) shouting, "My daughter got her period!" to your neighbor Lorainne, while watering your tulips; (2) wrapping up a stuffed shark with the message, "Looks like shark week came early;" and (3) throwing your daughter a period-themed brunch.

In the red plate's reflection, I saw feathered hair and black rubber bands encircling shiny braces. The rubber bands were meant to be Hot Topic-meets-braces. But it turns out that people mostly saw black olives. It also turns out that my mother had gone off the rails in her desire to be my personal cheerleader.

She had chosen #3—period brunch. Her desire to be supportive had finally overshadowed common sense.

In an effort to understand that my mother is not a crazy person, you must go back to the beginning. The details of my birth are hazy, except for an audio tape of my mother screaming and then, "It's a girl!" What was clear was that giving birth was a painful horror show that I never wanted to experience and that my mother was over the moon to finally get a daughter. Also, that audiotaping a birth is emphatically not the best way to highlight its joy. Together my mother and I shared ice cream cones, dreams, and the collective understanding that women were the best.

She made it her mission to get behind me in life. She was in my corner holding a sign that said, "You go, girl!" far before it was fashionable. When I showed a desire for reading, she bought every book Scholastic had to offer. I experienced every story about a girl who moves into a new neighborhood with only a wild horse to love. I read every *Misty of Chincoteague, Star of Montpelier*, and *Champ of Some Lonely, Mossy, Town with Too Many Birds*.

When I expressed a desire for drawing street art by placing flourishes on the walls of Living Room Street, she bought me countless art supplies. She is truly the most loving and supportive person you will ever meet. So supportive that she still has artwork like "Still Life with Macaroni" that I completed in the first grade. She also kept "Still Life with Macaroni 2 & 3," as well as "Moons Over Macaroni" in the tenth grade. At this point, I wonder if she just compulsively throws her bowl of macaroni-and-cheese in a bin labeled "Susie's Art." When I expressed a love of calligraphy, a kit magically appeared so that I could practice swirly lettering that I was convinced would garner much popularity in high school. My beautiful writing would not only earn me a place amongst the elite, but my handwritten letters would show whatever boy I liked that I was akin to Lady Diana. And now, she was here to support me as I crossed the threshold into womanhood. Would there be presents? I fearfully scanned the table.

I was twelve years old and not ready to celebrate the arrival of my Aunt Flo with my teenage brother, or dad, or anyone on the planet Earth. In fact, I would have rather eaten a cup of fermented dog food than have people find out. If no one EVER found out about this most embarrassing and gross thing, fine by me. The last thing I wanted was fanfare. Or a brunch. The inscription on the plate read, "Congratulations on your special day," but it might as well have read, "Just wanted to let everyone on planet Earth know that you are currently bleeding from your lady flower." Or "Did you guys watch *The Hunt for Red October*? It's actually happening on a micro level in Susie's pants right now." My mother thought that she had chosen a discreet path. When my older brother inquired about the crimson-themed waffle bar, she said, "Oh, that's private," as if somehow he would miss the crimson tide now creeping across my face.

As I painfully wolfed down strawberry waffles, one thing became clear. As a woman, I would have to endure countless indignities. My mother would not always take the right approach, but she would be there at each milestone. I would don the scarlet cloak of adulthood and become a spirited lady capable of great feats and able to fill a cone bra. I would hold my head high as my brother snickered under his breath. And I would never, EVER host a brunch. Period.

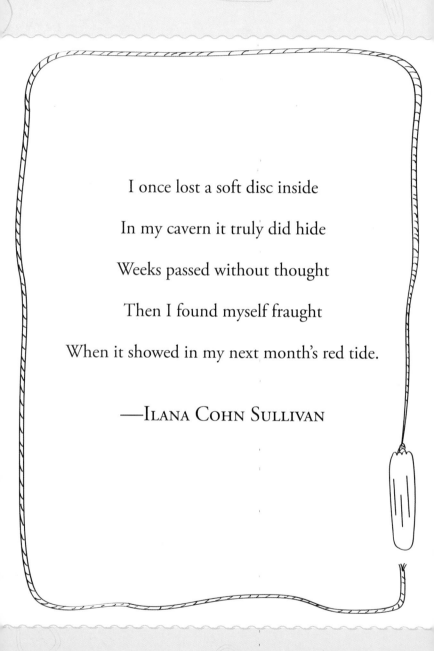

I once lost a soft disc inside

In my cavern it truly did hide

Weeks passed without thought

Then I found myself fraught

When it showed in my next month's red tide.

—Ilana Cohn Sullivan

TAMPONVISION

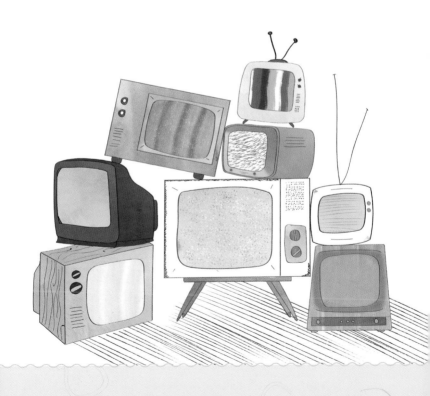

TAMPONVISION

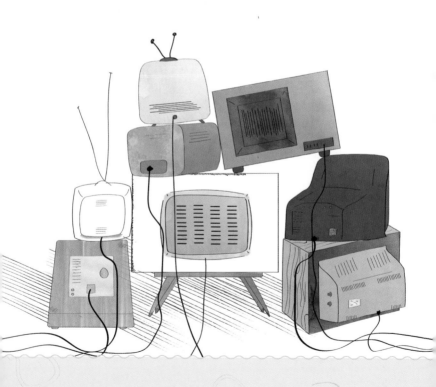

Menstruation can pop up in any media when you least expect it. And we love it. *Period. End of Sentence.* even won an Oscar! Below are some TV shows we found featuring the almighty period.

Better Things (Season 1, Episode 2)

Big Mouth (Season 1, Episode 2)

Black-ish (Season 4, Episode 6)

Blossom (Season 1, Episode 2)

Broad City (Season 3, Episode 10)

GLOW (Season 1, Episode 8)

Life & Beth (Season 1, Episode 1)

Mad Men (Season 5, Episode 12)

New Girl (Season 2, Episode 7)

Orange is the New Black (Season 4, Episode 5)

PEN15 (Season 2, Episode 5)

Starstruck (Season 1, Episode 1)

Sydney to the Max (Season 2, Episode 6)

The Middle (Season 3, Episode 2)

Yellowjackets (Season 1, Episode 5)

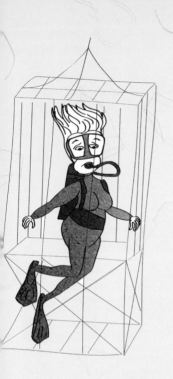

WORST PLACES
TO GET
YOUR PERIOD

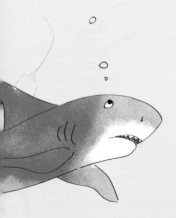

- Horseback riding on a first date
- Your bat mitzvah
- The deep end during a swimming party
- Volunteering at a dog pound
- A music festival in the woods with no bathroom in sight
- Testing taupe, white, or beige couches at a furniture shop
- Summer camp in a bunk surrounded by strangers
- On a pirate ship
- The top of the biggest water slide in Arlington, Texas
- Naked in a snowstorm
- On Labor Day at a white-pants party
- Inside a shark cage
- On top of a cheerleading pyramid
- Naked in a Korean spa while getting a skin scrub

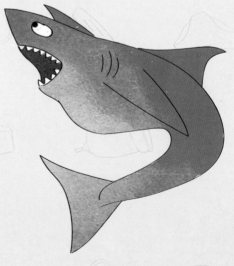

BEST PLACES TO GET YOUR PERIOD

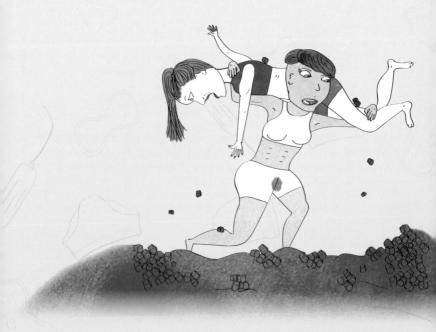

- On a color run

- Stomping on grapes to make wine

- While on a feminist retreat

- In a cherry Jell-O wrestling tournament

- Burning Man, next to the period art

- Women's March on Washington

- At a beat poetry event

- A photoshoot on top of a mound of rose petals

- La Tomatina festival in Spain

- While fertilizing your garden

- While dressed as Santa

- In a cozy cabin when you are expecting it

- While cosplaying in *Baywatch* outfits

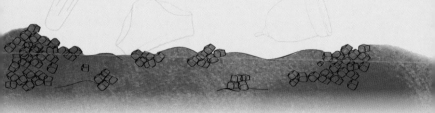

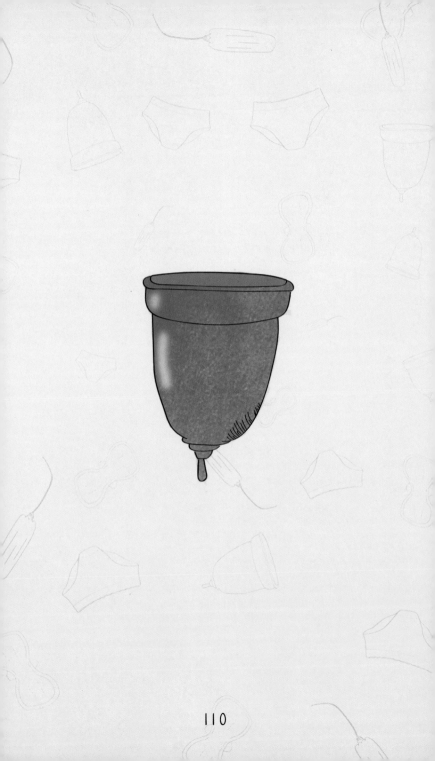

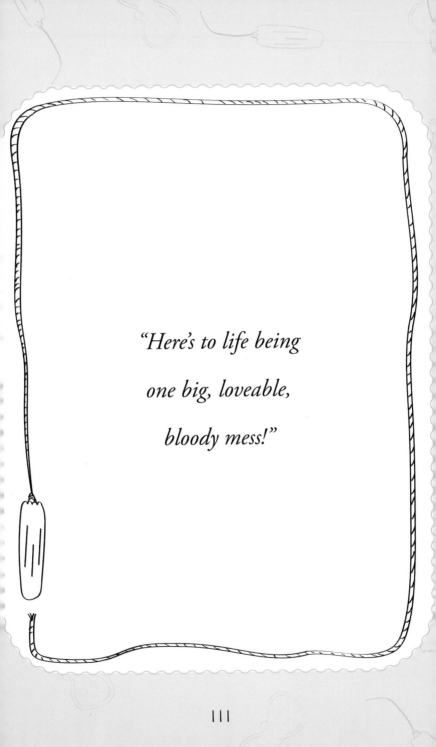

"Here's to life being

one big, loveable,

bloody mess!"

"ONE BIG BLOODY MESS"

By Steph Garcia

My periods growing up were a beast. I only got them, like, eight times a year, and they lasted two weeks or more at a time. They were heavy AF, and the cramps were so bad that all I wanted to do was stay lying down in the fetal position. On top of it, my mom was not into me using tampons so I used what she did: huge overnight pads. My period started at twelve years old, so there I was, a preteen, bleeding like I was dying with a brick between my legs trying to recite the periodic table by memory. (Hydrogen, helium, lithium, beryllium…)

Fast forward to college and my period symptoms escalated to include nausea and vomiting. #blessed. I finally went on birth control, and it felt like that moment in the movies where a light comes beaming through with an angel ready to save you. I finally had the period I always thought I was promised: regular, minimal cramping, NO vomiting! I was so diligent about taking my pill at the same exact time every day. I was liiiiiiiiiving, and I would do nothing to destroy it.

Except deciding to have a kid.

When my husband and I decided to try for our first kid, I was freaked out. Not about pregnancy or motherhood or all the actual things people freak out about. I was worried about going off birth control. What was this period going to be like?! Thankfully, I got pregnant quickly, had a fairly easy pregnancy, and, at the first possible moment postpartum, got back on a pill. However, newborn life is not favorable towards diligent pill taking. At least mine wasn't. So, I opted for an IUD.

And then came the discussion of kiddo numero dos.

Out came the IUD. A couple months after, I got my period and it stayed for over two weeks. I was like, "Oh, I got lucky that first time, but here it is. It's back with a vengeance. Cool cool cool." But I didn't think much of it.

I took an ovulation test, while still bleeding, and it came out positive. And then I started feeling a little weird, and cramping, and after a few days I turned to my husband and said, "I think I might be pregnant…" But I was still bleeding.

Three positive pregnancy tests later…

An addendum to this story is that I was meant to go on a weekend retreat in the middle of the woods with shoddy reception for a whole weekend. I had been looking forward to this retreat for months. I took the tests on Sunday night and was meant to leave on Friday of the same week for the retreat.

I wanted to confirm the home tests, so I called my OB-GYN Monday to schedule a blood test. The original blood test was scheduled for Friday, and I called them up again to move it to Wednesday so that maybe I could know by Friday for sure. I asked to rush my results, and the nurse was ALL about it when she heard about my retreat. I called the office Friday, and the front desk told me: "Congratulations! You're pregnant." I asked to talk to my doc because I was still bleeding, but she wouldn't be in until Tuesday.

I got ready for my retreat.

At two o'clock I got a phone call from another doctor in the office. I figured she got my message, and I said that I only had a couple questions. She stopped me. "Well, you ask me what—actually, let me just tell you what I was going to say." It was a bad start. I had one bite of a slice of pizza—it was the first thing I had eaten all day. I stopped eating and sat down on the floor of my kitchen.

She said a bunch of numbers: HCG levels were at 19,000 but should be at 5,000, progesterone levels should be 9 or 10 but mine were 4. It could be nothing, or it could be molar or ectopic or TWINS! I've never wished for twins so much in my life. And then I brought up the bleeding. And then I brought up the retreat. "Mmm. I would say either come in today for an ultrasound or stay near a hospital all weekend."

I went in for an ultrasound.

The ultrasound technician pulled up my uterus on the screen, pointed to what she called the "ring of fire," and said that it was all blood. I talked with a third doctor at the practice. (The one who called me wasn't even in the office! She had just been reviewing lab results and came across mine. Crazy. Anyway.) She asked me why I was even there. See, usually women don't go in until seven or eight weeks, but I was there incredibly early for no good reason, according to the charts. I was healthy, had a previously healthy pregnancy, etc. etc. etc.

This, however, was an ectopic pregnancy. I had an egg lodged in a fallopian tube. Which was causing the bleeding. That I thought was my period. Emergency surgery was scheduled for that evening.

So fast forward to a successful surgery and losing a fallopian tube. I called my doctor on Monday to check in, and her first question was not about how I was feeling or whether I was in pain. No. It was whether I had FOMO from missing the retreat. Which I took to mean she was not concerned about anything being wrong.

I was fortunate enough to get pregnant and have another baby. And since then, my periods have been everything I've wanted them to be, WITHOUT birth control! They're regular, minimal cramps and pains, and juuuuuust the right amount of blood. I don't know if it's the missing fallopian tube or the two kids, but I've finally learned to not despise my period and to listen to my body, instead of trying to suppress it. I'm not saying you have to lose body parts or grow humans to love your period. But our periods aren't our enemies, and there are so many new and innovative ways to make them manageable.

Here's to life being one big, loveable, bloody mess!

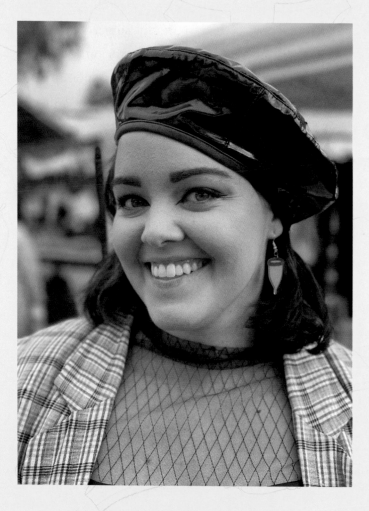

Art by Shelley Friedman (Model: Seneca Dykes)

"THE CANYON & THE RIVER"

By Laurissa Gold

"*Oh shi...........ttt!*" was all I could think of to say.

I was crouched behind a boulder at the bottom of the Grand Canyon on day two of a seven-day camping trip during spring break of my sophomore year of college.

This was not a reaction to the scenery around me. Nor was it in response to approaching wildlife. Instead, I was squatting out of sight, staring at the unmistakable stain in the crotch of my underpants, and panicking.

Getting one's period during a hiking trip is... pretty crappy. Getting it at the start of a week-long camping trip with a bunch of dudes, when you and your roommate are the only girls, is, frankly, traumatic. Beth and I had decided to "get away from it all" for vacation and signed up with the school's outdoor adventure club. We hadn't expected our group to consist of six super-fit, super-hot, nature-loving men, but we weren't complaining.

Little hitch: I was not anticipating my period and, more importantly, I was not prepared for my period. One would think that I would have had some idea of my cycle. Nope. I didn't see this coming at all. But there I was hiding in the brambles, crying into my panties, and trying to figure out a plan for the next five days of menstruation in a hot, sweaty desert without tampons or pads.

I did the best I could with the few thin squares of TP I had brought with me into the bush and headed back to camp. Once there, I rummaged through all the gear looking for any paper goods I could dedicate to the cause. That was when I realized that guys really don't use a lot of TP and they certainly don't bother bringing much when everything needs to be carried in their packs. Just my luck.

I considered mentioning the situation to Charlie, the hike leader, but I just couldn't bring myself to do it. Beth concurred. Unfortunately, I soon realized my problem was a bit more involved. The Grand Canyon is a very delicate ecosystem; it takes an eternity for things to break down in the arid climate, so everything you bring in with you, you must pack out (aside from natural body functions). All garbage, including used TP, went into the little brown paper bags we each carried around with us. Gross on a good day. Really off-the-charts nasty when you're having your period. Did I mention no tampons, and that it was really hot?

Luckily I dodged the cramps, the moodiness, and the exquisite pain of chocolate cravings and kept up with the group. No one but Beth knew my secret, though Charlie did give me much grief about how often I needed to duck into the bushes. On day four, we passed a group of hikers who told us coyotes had gotten into their camp a few nights back. They had strung their food up in a tree so nothing was eaten, but it was a scare nonetheless. Not the news I wanted to hear. I had been trying to be environmentally conscious and was still using my little brown bag, but I realized carrying around a significant amount of bloody waste paper was not the wisest move when in the midst of hungry animals with tremendous senses of smell. Beth suddenly—but not helpfully—recalled that menstruating women can give off pheromones that attract certain animals. This did not help the situation, though I secretly hoped that those "animals" might include some of the guys on the trip.

I couldn't decide what to do, but the longer I waited, the more stressed I got. I needed to commit to a decision: Bury my little bag of secrets in the dirt to throw wildlife off the scent (to heck with the environment) and hope it stayed buried. Stick my bag into the bottom of my pack and pray for the best. Or mortify myself by coming clean to Charlie to ask his advice and never be able to look him in the eyes again.

So, which did I do? Well, that's my secret; I'm not telling. I will say that we weren't ravaged by feral animals, the Grand Canyon survived and is still magnificent, and Charlie and I dated for a full year after the trip. So there is a happy ending after all. And from the moment I re-entered civilization I have never, ever left the house without being fully stocked with sanitary products. Lesson learned.

If you were stranded on a
deserted island on your period,
what would you do?

"SINGING IN THE RED"

By Malynda Hale

Singing on stage was where I belonged, and I knew it was what I wanted to do forever. I had wanted it since I was five years old, and any chance I got to perform for others was a dream come true. When I was in fifth grade, I got to perform my first solo in front of the school, and by the time I got to seventh grade, I was given more solos.

When I was eleven years old and in the seventh grade, a new kid arrived in school. He was kind and cute and loved performing as much as I did. A few weeks into his arrival, I had the biggest crush on him and I couldn't wait for him to hear me sing. If there was one thing I felt confident in at that age, it was that.

We had just been assigned solos for our upcoming spring show, and I was going to sing the female solo in "Seasons of Love" from the musical *Rent*. I couldn't have been more excited. I remember it like it was yesterday. It was more than just a regular day. It was even bigger than picture day. And I, being the genius that I was, decided to wear all white that day. White jeans, white shirt, white scrunchie (I'm clearly aging myself here). Why all white? I have no idea, but I would soon regret it.

When we were called into the choir room to rehearse the big number, my crush chose the seat behind me. I immediately felt butterflies. This was it. This was the big moment. Our music director asked us all to stand up and prepare to sing the song. The intro began, and the butterflies fluttered even more... but then they suddenly turned into a cramp. *That's weird*, I thought. *I've never felt that before*. And then it hit me at the exact moment I was about to sing my big solo...I just knew.

My period had suddenly made its grand entrance into my life. Of all the moments in the world to be shifted into womanhood, it had to be the day I wore all white and my crush was sitting behind me.

I got through the solo and everyone complimented me, including him. But afterward I pulled my shirt down over my butt and ran hysterically to the bathroom.

Lo and behold, a sea of red had flooded my underwear and seeped into my white jeans. Luckily my T-shirt covered enough of my pants, but I wanted nothing more than to go home.

I walked back into the classroom and told my teacher—who luckily was a female—and she excused me to the office.

I called my mom, and she picked me up. When I told her what happened, she cried. She couldn't believe her little girl was a woman now.

Meanwhile, all I could think was, *I wonder if he liked my voice?*

IF BROADWAY SHOWS WERE ABOUT PERIODS

Bled Misérables
Bloody Bloody Andrew Jackson
Bleed-a-ton (by Lin-Menses Miranda)
Cats (in Heat)
Annie Get Your Tampon
The Phantom of the Uterus
A Uterine Chorus Lining
Menses Mia!
My Fair Puberty
Padless in the Park
The Sound of Cramping
Pads and Dolls
Damn Menses
The Prom (When I Had My Period and Bled Through My Dress)
Once on This Lining
Hello, Flowy!
Into the Moods

"JUNIOR HIGH"

By Bekah Tripp

It was a cool, clear day in the Midwest. No indication of what was to come as I rode the bus to junior high. I sat there, in that yellow tin can of misunderstood youth, clutching my awkwardness to my fully blossomed, very early-in-the-game breasts, like a new momma holding a tiny babe she must tend to carefully, for at any moment the baby or the awkwardness might explode in a cacophony of the most hellish sounds ever heard by human ear and destroy the bearer of its enormous weight.

I digress. I disembarked from the bus and went to class, completely unaware. Completely. Unaware. That this day would be burned into my memory for the rest of my life and create a horrifying shared moment between my father and me that would and could only be paralleled by a second shared moment in which I sat next to said father in a movie theater some years later, at age sixteen, watching *From Dusk*

Till Dawn and listening to Cheech Marin talk about p*ssy for a solid forty-five seconds.

I digress, again. After one of my first classes of the day, it happened. I was alerted, on the sly, by a friend—nay, an ANGEL—that I had a large bright-red stain on the back of my light-wash denim jeans. Luckily, as a studied student of the '90s, I wore layers that day, and so I quickly tied a layer around my waist. I made a beeline for the nurse's office. I was incredibly embarrassed but managed to eek out that I had my period and had bled through my jeans and needed to call home.

***Sidenote: I must disrupt the train of thought to inform the reader regarding some key information. My father was a formidable man. He was 6'1", half Potawatomi Indian, and for most of my adolescent years, he rocked a mullet. It was real business in the front, never know if it's a good mood or bad mood party in the back. My father also worked as a supervisor for the post office and, for the majority of that time, worked nights. So follow those little bread crumbs—physically scary, moody, and his daytimes were reserved for his sacred sleep.

The above sidenote might give you some insight as to what a big deal this was: calling home. (And might

I also age myself by reminding you this was not the time of cell phones. I was also severely stressed by the thought that I might not catch my mom at work or rouse my dad at home...and then I'd be stuck all Carrie at the prom down my backside for the rest of the day at school.) In fact, I did not call home. I called my mother at work. Hoping and praying that she would leave and come rescue me. Do we think that happened? No. I know you didn't. You're fully buckled in and you get that a shit show unfoldeth before you. So I reach my mom and beg and plead and though she loves me more than life, she simply can't leave work...and she rings my dad. She manages to wake the sleeping giant and I'm alerted, at some point, that he's on his way.

"On his way" is relative as I was bussed to the far end of the district and so the commute was about twenty minutes or so. A *LONG* twenty minutes. I wait. I wait some more. It's agony. FINALLY, I am alerted to the fact that my father has dropped off some pants at the front office, and I make my way from the nurse's office to my nice, clean, who-knows-what-the-hell-my-father-grabbed-to-bring-to-me-at-school pants. True to form, they are not cute, they are a little snug, and I sincerely do not even recognize the abomination of pants sitting before me. But they are blood-less, and as such, they are acceptable. I go to the bath-room, the hellmouth of the public school building, change, and head back to class.

Do NOT unbuckle your safety belt. This ride isn't over yet. The Universe was not done with me this day!! A mere hour after my return to the doldrums of middle school, another angel finds me in the hallway as I zombie walk to the next class and subtly notes that I have a…large…bright…red…stain on the back of my pants. Nope. This is not a drill. It happened a second time.

At this point, I've had my fill and I am just beside myself. I head back to the nurse's office and their sur-prise in seeing me again so soon was only outdone by my mortified shell of a soul, which now feels the mounting weight of having to disturb my father…a second…time. Which I do. Or rather, I have my mother do. At this point, I'm sure she's ready to aban-don work and come to my aid, but it wouldn't be fast enough. I mean, nothing can possibly whisk me away from this nightmare of a day at a speed that would be sufficient, but my father can end this journey into future therapy sessions faster than she and so she calls him, again.

It is a long wait. Longer than before, it seems. I'm finally called from the nurse's office to the front office. My father is there. We don't speak other than for me to ever so coolly and in my bravest voice say, "Thanks, Dad." We get in the car, we drive home. I head straight to my bedroom then the bathroom to change. I cry a bit. I wait for my mom to come home. And then, it's on to the next day.

I wish it had ended with perhaps a donut waiting for me in the car on that second pick-up. Some small token from my dad to express that he understood what a dignity-shredding day this had been. That would have been a fun and upbeat ending. But I never promised that, dear reader. He wasn't that kind of dad.

But all is not lost! I got a great story out of it, I can buy my own donuts now when I need a bit of comfort, and it turns out that this was a clue on the road to my endometriosis diagnosis eight years later. And this, this defining moment in my life, made me stronger and a hell of a lot more resilient, because no matter what, I survived bleeding through two sets of boss ass denim, in junior high, and no one can take that away from me. That kid was brave As Fuck, and I'm damn proud of her.

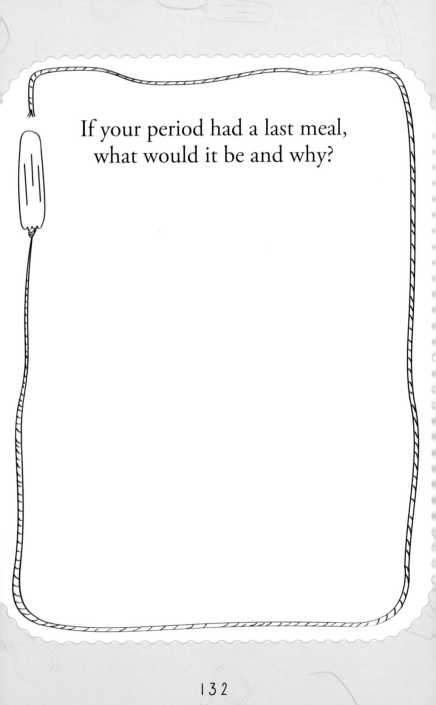

If your period had a last meal,
what would it be and why?

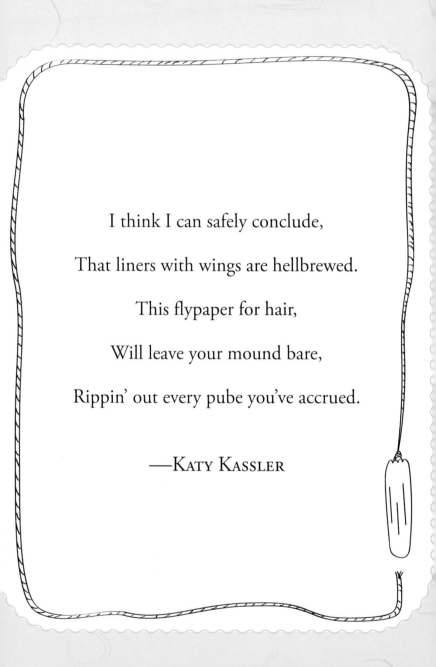

I think I can safely conclude,

That liners with wings are hellbrewed.

This flypaper for hair,

Will leave your mound bare,

Rippin' out every pube you've accrued.

—Katy Kassler

"WHEN ON MY PERIOD, SHOULD I...?"

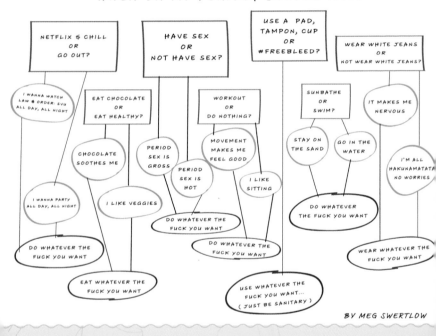

BY MEG SWERTLOW

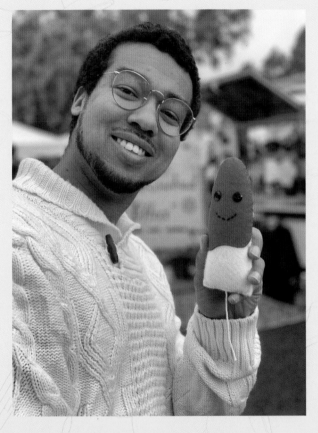

Art by Shelley Friedman (Model: Brennon Dixson)

"DEAR DAUGHTER"

By Amanda Hirsch

Dear daughter,

You love to talk to me, just like I loved to talk to my mother when I was little. Me being on the toilet does not dim your passion. Oh, the conversations we've had with me on the can! Often, I've spoken to you not as myself, but while impersonating a favorite character of yours; we call this "character time." I'll pretend to be Twilight Sparkle from *My Little Pony*, or Bart Simpson, and you'll tell me (them) all about yourself, offer them advice, and imagine how they might react to all the ways in which your life and world are different from theirs.

But when I have my period? The party's over. You recoil. "You're peeing blood!!" you yell, as you flee the room—as if running from a fire. As if running for your life.

Shield your eyes, Twilight. Look away, Bart. Run, daughter, run!

On the one hand, I want to tell you, and them, "This is natural, this is nothing to be afraid of. It's part of the amazing superpower that women's bodies have, to grow babies inside of us, should we want to do that someday."

But, of course, that's bullshit.

It's true, but (and), also, it's bullshit.

If I could press a magic button, my dear daughter, and save you and every single girl on earth, even the cartoon ones, even the ones with unicorn horns and Pegasus wings, from ever having to have your period, I would.

Why would I wish upon you the blood, the hormonal stew? The headaches (migraines, for the women in our family); the tense neck, shoulders, and back; the sore hip? The diarrhea, the fatigue, and worst of all, the depression? Every month, the heaviness sets in; I swim upstream to feel hopeful, energized.

Does getting to have a baby after months and years of this make it "all worth it"?

I honestly don't know. What kind of a monster would I be if I said you weren't "worth it"? And yet, how can I honestly say that the pain, depletion, and disruption my menstrual cycle has caused was something I would willingly choose if given the choice, no matter how transcendent the prize, twenty-plus years later? Especially when that transcendence is intermingled with its own pain, depletion, and disruption?

I think you know that I spent a long time thinking that I didn't want to become a mother. What you don't know, because I've never elaborated, because that would be inappropriate, is why: I saw brilliant women turn into slaves to their children. No more hobbies, passions, or personal interests, just sippy cups, Cheerios, and sleepless nights. I saw kids screaming in restaurants. I thought, "I will not have what she's having." (One day you'll watch *When Harry Met Sally* and you will get this reference.)

Then, in my early thirties, I held a dear childhood friend's newborn to my chest, and something awakened. Hormones surged. Suddenly, motherhood became irresistible. It strikes me now, writing this, that it's as if my body was in cahoots against me the whole time, gaslighting me: first, making me bleed/ hurt/see the world through bleak-colored glasses, and then, making me want the thing that the suffering was all in service of—all while my brain said, "Really? Motherhood? That looks kind of like a pain in the ass."

My dear daughter, let me be honest with you: motherhood *is* a pain in the ass.

It is a deeply painful and wrenching experience. And, what is also true, is that you are joy. And my love for you could light up the sky.

If you ever become a mother, you will confront these same seemingly contradictory truths, or your own version of them. Maybe, like me, you will come to understand things thus: that it is possible to adore your child without adoring the job of being a mother or the havoc it wreaks on your identity. That sometimes you are in the mood for the job, and sometimes you are not because of how it eats into your time to do the things you want to do, the thoughts you want to think, the conversations you want to be having… not about your child's favorite cartoon characters but about, you know, *Ted Lasso*, and the meaning of life.

And maybe, like me, you'll come to believe that as destabilizing and stressful as motherhood can be, its very difficulty can become a gift—a long lesson in confronting self, and deciding how you want to be in this world (not a fun process, but a meaningful and enriching one).

But first, you'll bleed.

Now, you've told me that you do not plan to give birth and that it sounds horrible. I hasten to clarify, I have barely described the experience of childbirth to you, but what little you've gleaned has been enough to make your incredibly sharp young mind tell you, "No thanks, not for me." Instead, you plan to adopt—a seven-year-old, no less, so you can avoid the intense labor (pun intended) of the early years. A girl. So that someday, you too can write a letter about "peeing blood."

Of course, you are nine. You are in the fourth grade. You may change your mind many times over before such decisions move from theoretical to immediate. And even if you don't change your mind of your own free will, then, as my own story makes clear, your body may change it for you.

If your hormones take the wheel, I'm sorry for you to discover the ways in which you are not in control of your choices—but then, I guess having your period every month (give or take), year after year, will prepare you for your body to have its way.

I see now, writing this letter to you, how, in this patriarchal world that oppresses women, our own bodies oppress us first, by enslaving us to our birth function. Even if we have contraceptives. Even if we have the power, despite strong opposition, to choose to terminate a pregnancy. We are still in bodies that are in so many ways primed to not only make, but also to want babies.

And yet. And yet, amidst the rage I so clearly feel at these hormonal afflictions of womanhood, and the ways in which they encroach on my sense of freedom, I must also admit that somewhere in this stew of feelings is an acknowledgement that my body is not just a tyrant. It is also an integral part of me. I may strain to make it subservient to the wishes of my mind, but that way of being denies the body's own intelligence, the stories it holds, the power it contains.

What if my body didn't gaslight me into wanting motherhood? What if it was expressing something I truly wanted but that my mind could not comprehend? Are the body's desires less legitimate than the mind's?

I should pause here and point out, in the spirit of teaching you media literacy and discernment, that I'm generalizing womanhood based on my personal experience. Which is bad journalism, but fair game, I'd say, in a letter from a mother to her daughter. Still, you should know that, of course, not all women become moms. Their hormones don't cast a spell, or they resist the spell. Or, on the other hand, many women want to get pregnant but cannot. So of course my experience is just that: my experience.

But you're in my genetic lineage. So the chances are decent that my experience will, at least somewhat, predict yours. Further back in your lineage, my own mother didn't think she wanted to have kids, either, but then decided: "I get my period every month, I might as well see what this thing I'm primed for is all about." Was it really an intellectual process for her, or was she rationalizing the tug of hormones?

Does it matter? Ultimately, whether our mind chooses something or our body does—is one more legitimate than the other? Two branches are part of the same tree.

My dad wanted children, "because that was what people did," so that was another factor in my mom's decision—unlike in my case, where your father wanted children about as much as Bart Simpson wants to do homework.

Yeah, that little.

Of course, now he loves you as much as Twilight Sparkle loves her friends, and then some.

A witchy friend of mine says some people believe that when we have our periods, we're in our full power.

I sure don't feel powerful, as I bleed through another pair of underpants, while trying to overcome intense sadness. Then again, the blood is a reminder of my body's ability to make life. If my menstrual cycle didn't hurt so much, I could see celebrating it as a monthly reminder of my creative power.

Maybe it's a monthly reminder that power comes with a price?

A woman I know has a company that helps women founders align their menstrual cycles with their businesses, so they're productive at the times of the month when they have the most energy, and can rest when they need to. This is clever and also names what we avoid saying, which is that menstruation is a disability. It disables us, for some period of time, every single month (give or take). It limits us. Every woman learns to live with this disability.

Or, another interpretation: our bodies are not in a consistent state of being. We ought to live our lives in ways that honor that, instead of demanding or denying our needs in service of capitalist consistency.

It all comes down to this, baby: I don't know what to tell you, when you run from the bathroom, away from me "peeing blood." Run while you can? You can't outrun the inevitable? There might be layers of meaning and potential value to be discerned from this undeniably painful aspect of womanhood? Being a woman is hard? But oh, my god, the power we are capable of, and how I hope that in your lifetime, the world will ease up in its efforts to dim women's power and that you will never let the world dim yours?

That sisterhood is essential to your salvation, so find you a community of girls, and later, women, who have your back, and who will see you and hear you and support you? Find yourself doctors and other healers, too, who will respectfully partner with you in tending to your health, every aspect of it, and help your well-being shine?

Or maybe, in the beginning, just this: I love you, no matter what. I am here for you, no matter what.

And as you navigate the complexities of identity and womanhood, know that I don't have all the answers—but for you, my dear, sweet daughter, I will sit on a toilet and pretend to be Bart Simpson, over and over again, even before I've had my morning tea.

Love,

Mommy

My daughters are the best people ever

We have a bond that no one can sever

But every month I do cheer,

My period is here!

No more kids, not now, no, never.

—JESSICA GLASSBERG

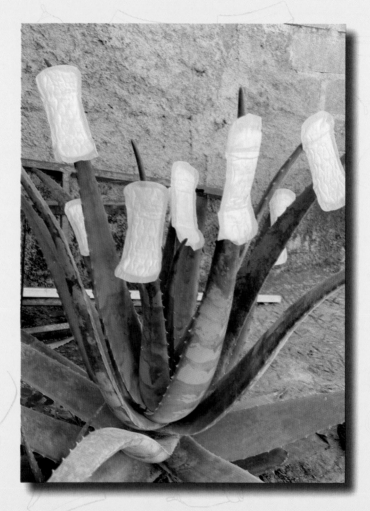

Photo by Neno

SLANG FOR PERIODS

Call it what you like.
We sure do.

Aunt Flo

Bloody Sunday

On the Rag

Happy Hemorrhage

Red Evacuation

Bloody Show

My Exclamation Point

Moon Cycle

My Cycle

Shedding Uterine Lining

Monthly Visitor

The Hunt for Red October

Shark Week

Surfing the Crimson Wave

The Red Sea

Murder Scene

Closed for Business

Riding the Cotton Pony

Red Menace

Not Preggers

My "Don't F*ck with Me" Week

Red Tide

The Big Show

Menses

Carrie's Prom Day

Time to Bring the Dark Pants

Mommy Needs Chocolate Week

Vampire's Feast

Crime Scene

Crampville

The Sloughening

Underwear Killer

My Moon

Cramp City

Murderville

Biology

First Blood

Blood Bath

Lady Time

Monthly Visitor

Mess Under the Dress

Flooded Undies
Bleedy Grossy
My Lady
My Own Red Tent
Girl's Week

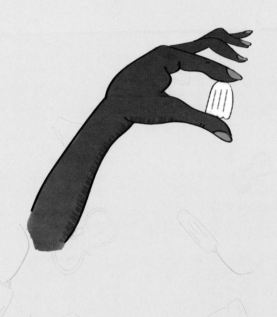

"SHOW ME THE MONEY"

By Dani Adaliz

There's a saying: acting is reacting. There's no quicker reaction than when you're on your way to a big audition…and you happen to get your period.

Before I left my place to head out, I had been waiting for my period to let down. It felt like I had that ball of period kind of waiting at the, like, bottom of my uterus, ready to release. I peed, I pooped, I sneezed, I coughed (I had a cold). Nothing was happening. It felt stuck. So, I left thinking it would hold up until I got back.

I hadn't had any time to buy pads or tampons. I figured I could do that after, but then there was so much traffic. I mean there's never not traffic in LA, especially on the 405, which is exactly the highway I had to drive on.

My agent, Laura, was not sympathetic.

"Dani, you're late already. You have to hurry up when you get there."

(Which actually makes no sense. Hurry up when I get there? I'm trying to hurry now, no?)

"Dani, don't be late! This is a lot of money! I need this money! You need this money!"

The pressure was on. Not just to book the job but to actually get to the audition on time.

My cold was also not sympathetic because as I hung up the phone, I took the biggest sneeze and just the gush of first blood came all over my white and green Totoro spandex pants. There was no way to hide it. I had to call Laura back.

"What?"

"…I sneezed and I got my period all over my pants?"

"Dani! How does this happen?? How do you not know when you get your period! Are you fourteen?!"

She was just repeating, "Are you fourteen?" at me like the answer would change. Hey, maybe I could *play* fourteen. I can't play fourteen, but what could I do? I was stuck in traffic and covered in blood! Maybe she could tell them I had an emergency?

"Dani! They will not wait! You must go now!"

By this time, I had pulled off and found a place to buy pants, which I told Laura. She calmed down a bit.

"Okay. I will hold them off. But you better do a good audition damnit."

I walked in with my sweater around my waist, and after buying a pair of pants, I searched for the bathroom. I stopped a woman employee who took one look at me and let out a weird, confused "…Oh, no."

She led me to the bathroom and just kept repeating things like "Oh, no… Oh, man… Oh, my… Oh, no." Those comments don't really say anything but also say EVERYTHING. She was judging, for sure.

Well, on top of all this, I had the period poops. I was stuck in this department store restroom, with some great period-free pants, and I had to wait it out on the toilet.

TEXT FROM LAURA: HOW LONG DOES IT TAKE TO CHANGE YOUR PANTS?! IS THERE A BIG LINE?! WHAT IS HAPPENING?!

I calmly texted back, *"I have diarrhea now."*

I've never felt closer to my agent as I did in that moment.

I finally got to the audition, cleaned up, tampon in, pooped out. I felt alright about myself. The audition itself was meant to be emotional: I had to cry, my husband just died, great. I was completely in that emotional state already! The casting director looked at me.

"Can you think of anything, like, sad that may have happened to you to get into it?"

"Yeah. I'm on my period."

Silence. She stared at me with a look that felt like she thought I was the most disgusting human being she had ever encountered. Instantly, I started crying so hard because I felt so judged.

And I got a callback!

But I also ruined my favorite pants. *My Neighbor Totoro* will never be the same.

If your period was a celebrity, who would it be and why?

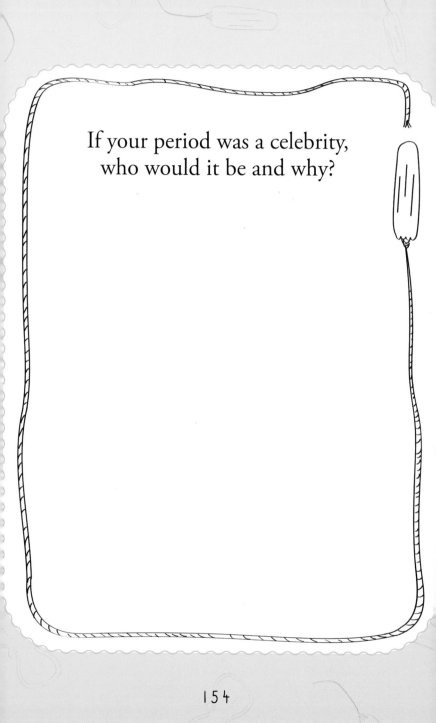

"PERIODS NO MORE"

By Grace Kestler

The first time I thought I had my period was actually a false alarm. (It was a UTI on Christmas Day!) In fact, I don't even remember the start of my real period, because the first memory has been stuck in my head. But I do remember how my period became a monthly burden. Not because I had horrible cramps or an extra heavy flow, but because it made me hyperaware of my physical disability.

I use a wheelchair, cannot stand at all, and have very limited dexterity in my hands due to having muscular dystrophy. Because of this, it was basically impossible to use tampons. I'm assuming tampons were invented to help women go about more of their normal lives during their period. When I was younger, the biggest thing I noticed was not being able to swim when I was on my period. So, a tampon would have been nice.

Pads caused their own issues, as they often got stuck together before I got them in position… and then I had to successfully shimmy my underwear up while sitting on the toilet (remember I can't stand). This didn't work every time. And because I'm such a thrifty gal, I cursed at throwing away fifty cents before it even got used.

Like all things in life…I got used to it. I was that girl who packed five extra-long pads with wings for a night out. Bad fingers are one thing, but bad drunk fingers were a whole new challenge level.

When I started taking birth control, I realized this created an opportunity to skip my periods. Finally, I could gain some control back. I could skip if I knew I'd be on vacation or was planning to go swimming. Or maybe just a really hot week of summer where I didn't want to deal with sitting on a bumpy pad all day in the heat!

Fast forward to my early thirties, and I actually don't have a period now. I decided to get an IUD. One of the biggest reasons I made this choice was that I had heard that in some women their periods would completely stop. I was lucky enough to be one of them. The consistency of birth control was also a nice perk.

(Oh, am I implying that disabled women have sex? Yes, indeed I am!)

Aside from the initial, excruciating pain from placing the IUD, it has changed my life. No more frustrating pads to deal with. It's funny though— sometimes I miss my period. As it's a clear sign that I'm not pregnant. While it wouldn't be the end of the world, pregnancy while living with a disability is a challenge I'm just not sure I'm ready for. I'm not sure if I'll ever be ready. For now, I'm happy saving a few bucks a month not having to buy pads and swimming on any hot summer day!

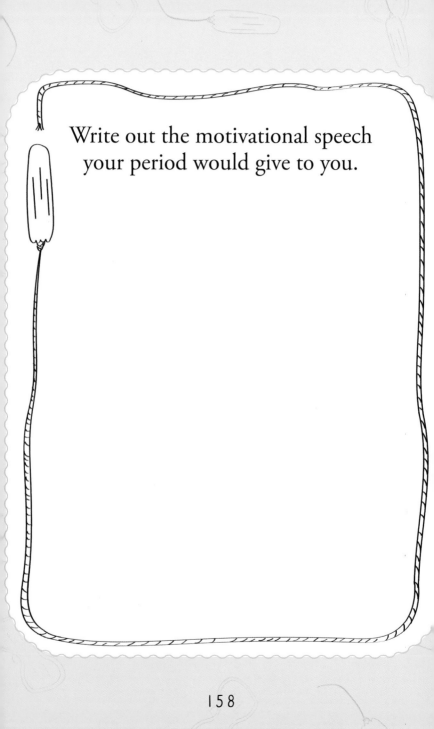

Write out the motivational speech
your period would give to you.

"ENDOMETRIOSHIT"

By Madeleine Hernandez

Remember how, at the dawn of modern medicine, women who were sick or complained of any ailment were diagnosed as "nervous," "crazy," or a "witch"? I think the modern equivalent is when doctors begin any visit by asking for the date of your last period and then handing you a "How Depressed Are You?" worksheet. Clearly, our experiences must be questioned if we're pregnant, on our period, or chemically imbalanced. But if we're not pregnant, not on our period, and not experiencing a mental crisis, we...still must have our experiences questioned. Being a woman in pain SUCKS. Zero stars. Would not recommend.

Thankfully, when women know they're not alone in an experience, they are empowered to advocate for themselves and each other. The #MeToo movement is one example but so are mom groups, survivor support groups, and, in my personal experience, the community of women (and men!) afflicted with endometriosis.

My period arrived two months before my fifteenth birthday. It was terribly irregular, often catching me off guard. If I didn't have access to a pad or tampon, I would resort to the classic "wad of toilet paper in panties" move. Day one was always the worst, call-out-of-work-miss-events-can't-eat-worst. Heavy bleeding and cramps so intense that I would usually fall asleep from pain exhaustion before any medicine could kick in. If I didn't time the meds right, then I'd get jolted awake screaming at 4 a.m., which is not great when you're spending the night at your new boyfriend's place and he thinks you're dying. My period lasted a full seven days; and on day five, when it would look like it was ending and I had the audacity to wear a mere panty liner, I would be hit by a truck of pain. These were different from the cramps I'd get at the beginning of my cycle—they came out of nowhere and knocked the air out of me. I call them "dry cramps," because it kind of feels like blood is being wrung out of a dry cotton ball of nerves. I don't know how else to describe it.

I remember sitting in my high school sophomore AP English class, doubled over, sweating, wincing, holding my breath while the lower half of my body writhed in pain, hot blood filling my giant pad. I started getting cervical spasms. I couldn't wear underwear or leggings with a seam down the middle because it felt like getting stabbed in the crotch. When I was out of college and performing at a theme park, I stood in photos with kids as pain shot down my legs, enveloping my back, and grating my uterus. In between photos, I doubled over in pain, catching my breath, knees shaking, willing myself to stand up straight so that I wouldn't get in trouble, thankful that the heavy character head kept my pained face hidden from the public. On days like that, I would visit the on-site physical therapists and, if one of my friends was working, they'd let me lay down on one of the treatment tables on my break with the lights off, a peel-and-stick heat patch intended for someone's neck stuffed between my swollen belly and the band of my underwear. I was at the Getty Villa in Los Angeles on a date as cramps throbbed through my pelvis and legs, requiring me to sit down every five minutes from the pain and exhaustion. I had to leave a friend's wedding shower early because the 600 mg of Advil I'd taken didn't stop the pain that brought me to tears and made it difficult to walk. Sex felt like sharp fingernails or

161

burning along my cervix. My intestines cramped from bowel movements.

Every doctor said my experience wasn't special and my pain was considered part of "normal cramps" (dysmenorrhea, if you're fancy). They all suggested going on birth control if I couldn't "handle the pain," but I never felt comfortable with that option. When I was a virgin, they said that Pap smears made me yelp in pain because I hadn't had sex yet (to the male doctor who said that: kindly get fucked); and when I was finally getting my sex on, they said my cervical and vulvar pain was from not having *enough* sex (to those female doctors: join the circus, CLOWNS). And I believed all of it because they're doctors! We're told to trust them! I didn't know anyone else who experienced what I was going through; and if they were going through it, they weren't talking about it.

In January of 2017, I noticed a sharp pain on the right side of my lower abdomen. I would occasionally experience painful ovulation, so I assumed as much. But it lasted for three months. Then I started having back spasms and I couldn't wear clothes that were tight around my waist. So, that May, I had ultrasounds done, thinking maybe I had a swollen appendix or something. I'd be just like Madeline in the books! Except my name is spelled correctly (do not come for me).

At the follow-up appointment, the nurse practitioner—who was leagues better than any of the GPs I had there—explained that they had found an endometrioma (aka "chocolate cyst" for the dark fluid it contains, which is highly toxic and not, like I had hoped, an au naturel hot fudge) on my right ovary; and at ten cm, it was the size of an infant's head and needed to be removed. She said it was likely that I had endometriosis considering all of my symptoms. But I wasn't so sure. After all, no doctor had ever brought it up as a possibility, and my friends with endometriosis seemed to have intense symptoms like frequent bleeding and constant debilitating pain. I only had symptoms during my period. As I would later learn, there are several markers that appear in most patients: intense period pain, heavy periods, and pelvic floor dysfunction. But mostly, it was the endometrioma. Apparently it's a dead giveaway.

Now that I had a name for what I was going through, I could get treatment, right? LOL. No. This, dear reader, is where I had to both educate and learn to advocate for myself.

A friend told me about a Facebook group called Nancy's Nook, a research hub for people with endometriosis. They are not a support group; their whole reason for existing is to empower patients to advocate for the treatment they deserve. It was a game changer. They had links to the most current published research on endometriosis, and to sites of the surgeons who specialized in excision surgery—the gold standard for endo treatment—where they took the time to debunk long-held and dangerous models of diagnosing, treating, and talking about the disease. Nancy (a retired nurse and actual real person) even had a list of questions to take to potential doctors and a database of surgeons she personally contacted to ensure they were abiding by the latest research. Women were posting their personal experiences—most of them so similar to mine in both symptoms and lack of medical intervention. Everything I thought I knew about this chronic disease was wrong. I spent weeks just reading and connecting the dots. I had been sick since I was fifteen. On average, it takes seven to twelve years for women to get diagnosed. It took me seventeen years.

I was referred to a gynecologist who confirmed endometriosis due to "fused organs" (her words). Did you know all of your guts should be easily movable when a doctor is fist-deep in you? I did not. She referred me to an oncologist-gynecologist for surgery but said that after surgery I'd need to get pregnant immediately because "I didn't have much time and it was a good way to treat the disease." That doctor said that after ablation surgery (laser burning), her treatment plan would be to put me into early menopause for three months via a class D drug and then for me to immediately have a baby, because she believed that was the only way to "manage" endometriosis, *AND* since she believed the only way to cure it was with a full hysterectomy, it was important that I have a baby first. I was thirty-two years old.

Let's start with the obvious audacity here: having a baby is a life choice, not a fucking treatment plan. There is an unsettling focus in women's healthcare on popping out babies instead of ensuring we can have normal, pain-free lives. Yes, endometriosis has a high chance of infertility, but still, CAN WE LIVE??

Thankfully, I had done my reading. I learned that a hysterectomy can ONLY be a cure if a patient is diagnosed with a separate condition known as adenomyosis. The class D drug is so dangerous you're not supposed to be on it for more than three months at a time because it can destroy your body, but you have doctors out here prescribing it from six months to multiple years. Finally, ablation surgery is to endometriosis what cutting off the top of a rotting tooth is to a cavity; it doesn't get to the root of the problem.

Next to research, the most important part of self-advocacy is documentation. You gotta document E V E R Y T H I N G. Case in point: the Onc-Gyn I was referred to was actually a specialist in ovarian cancer. After asking her all of my questions, she outright said, "I'm not an endometriosis specialist." I asked her if she would please write that in her report notes, and she agreed. What I was doing was building a case for my shitty HMO insurance to let me see the only surgeon in my area at the time who specialized in endo excision surgery. I had already submitted a request for a consultation and been summarily denied. He was out of network, and there was no institutional understanding of his expertise. But when my insurance got the report from the non-specialist, it was approved. And let me tell you, after meeting with the excision specialist that July, I wept in the parking lot. It was a combination of sheer relief, finally being validated, and finally knowing that I would be safe with this medical professional. Even so, shitsurance (new word alert!) sent me back to that Onc-Gyn. So I amped myself up for that appointment and brought my partner at the time for support. I was dead set on not leaving until I got that goddamn referral. The doctor walked in, confused why I was there. Frustrated by having her time wasted, she asked, "Do you want to have surgery with me or with this surgeon you found?" "The surgeon," I replied. A beat. "Okay, I'll write it down in my notes." I looked at my partner—what just happened?

On December 4, three days before my scheduled surgery, I got a call from my insurance rep telling me that the surgery had been approved. Reader: I wept.

The surgery went extremely well. I was officially diagnosed with stage IV endometriosis and DIE (deep infiltrating endometriosis), which has a high rate of recurrence. I don't think I'm "cured," but I am able to function like a human person. Another thing I advocated for was pelvic floor therapy. The pelvic floor gets so fucked when you have endo and uber fucked when you have abdominal surgery; but I'm proud to report, almost a year and a half after I started therapy, I was able to have pain-free sex for the first time. Reader: I wept. Again.

Mine can be considered a success story, if being alive on this rapidly deteriorating earth in a declining society can be seen as successful, but I'm still angry. I'm angry at medical racism, sexism, and biases that keep people under the thumb of their pain. Pain that their doctors could help identify if only they listened instead of questioned, or looked for answers as hard as they found excuses. I'm angry that a disease that affects every one in ten women in this day and age is still so poorly understood and researched that even board-certified gynecologists don't understand the basics. I'm angry that one of my best friends was escorted out of her doctor's office by the wrist because she was crying from frustration and pain. I'm angry that Aubrion Rogers, a thirty-year-old Black woman, died in January of 2022 from a ruptured cyst that was caught months earlier but not removed for reasons unknown even to herself. Something like death from an untreated yet diagnosed problem is likely rooted in medical racism, with Black women receiving the worst of it.

I'm angry, but I am not alone. None of us are. And none of us are powerless, even in the midst of debilitating pain and mistreatment. When we trust ourselves, listen to our bodies, educate ourselves, practice self-advocacy, and share our experiences with others, we create space for more people to do the same. That is what leads to change.

(But if you're angry like me: welcome to the team. Let's fuck shit up.)

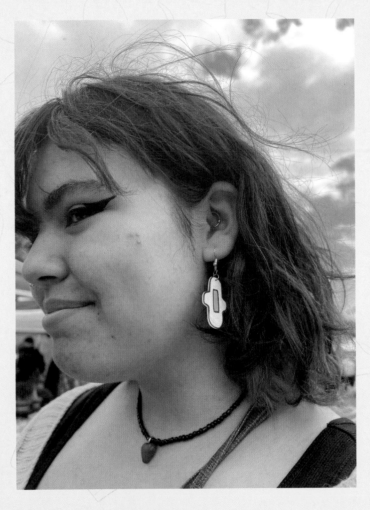

Art by Shelley Friedman (Model: Zurie Cobb)

PERIODS

OF THE

W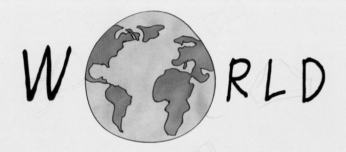RLD

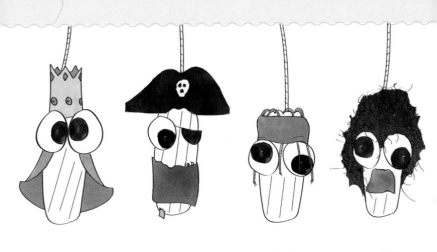

SWEDEN: A Swedish children's public service channel aired a video in 2015 called "The Period Song" featuring dancing tampons with googly eyes to help educate kids on periods. Hooray for periods!

IRELAND: Grocery chain Lidl announced in 2021 that customers could claim one free box of pads or tampons each month from their stores.

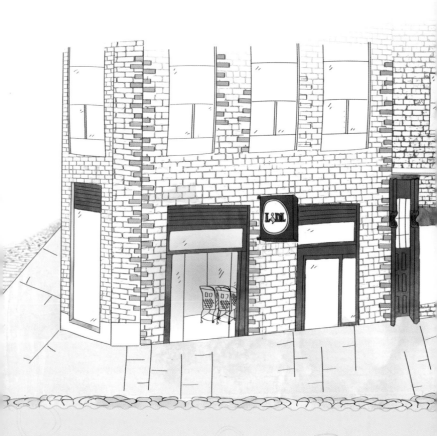

SCOTLAND: In 2020, Scotland passed a bill that made period products—such as tampons and pads—free to all who need them.

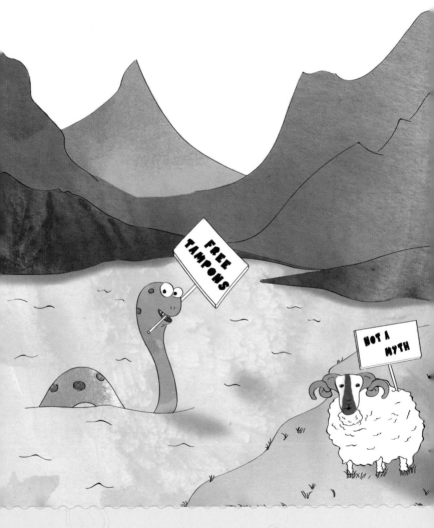

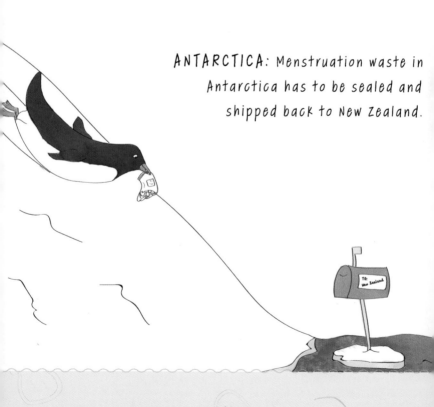

ANTARCTICA: Menstruation waste in Antarctica has to be sealed and shipped back to New Zealand.

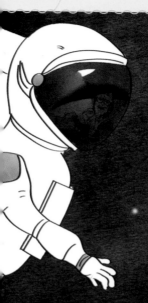

SPACE: Getting your period in space isn't dangerous! But some astronauts find it inconvenient and prefer to suppress their periods while there.

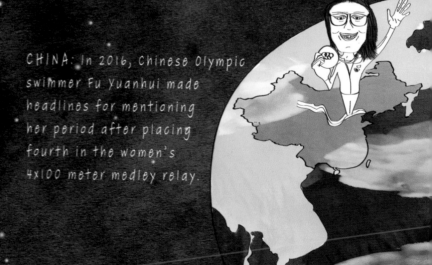

CHINA: In 2016, Chinese Olympic swimmer Fu Yuanhui made headlines for mentioning her period after placing fourth in the women's 4x100 meter medley relay.

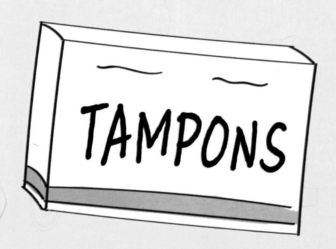

JOKES! JOKES! PERIOD JOKES!
With Kristine Kimmel & Jessie Gaskell

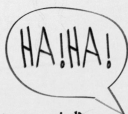

How do you know if you're about to start your period?

WHY WOULD YOU SAY THAT HOW DARE YOU ASK ME THAT IS SO DISRESPECTFUL—

How many tampons does it take to screw in a lightbulb?

One, but now you've ruined the light socket.

What's black and white and red all over?

My underwear when I'm wearing a menstrual cup.

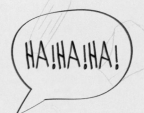

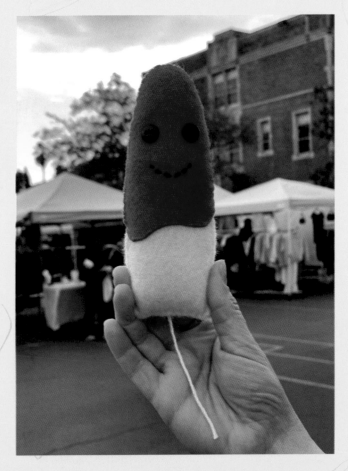

Art by Shelley Friedman

"THE SCREENING ROOM"

By Amy Albert

It was happening. My big break. Things were happening fast. Just a few months earlier, a director approached me after a show I performed in as a character named Delilah Dix, a boozy, pill-popping lounge singer who sits atop a piano and regales the audience with tales of debauchery. The director, we'll call him Cal, explained that he was making a documentary focusing on three early television comedians, including the brilliant comic actress Martha Raye. Cal said that Delilah Dix "smacks a bit of Martha" and asked if I could come out to LA to shoot some segments. Fast forward a few days and I am on the red-eye to LA, and my body is buzzing with excitement. I couldn't sleep thanks to the nonexistent leg room and the cramps churning around my lower abdomen that I chalked up to my nerves. I hadn't gotten many details about the filming. In fact, I hadn't asked a single question.

179

And an hour after landing, I pulled my rental, a puce hatchback, in front of a beautiful, huge house owned by the creator of a very successful sitcom, who we'll call Bill.

Admittedly, after living in 250-square-foot shitholes in New York for eight years, I would've been impressed with any dwelling where the bathroom and kitchen were separated. But this place *really* was a mansion, and it was awesome. In hindsight, I probably made too big a deal of it. I openly gawked at the place, and I'm pretty sure Bill heard my clumsy "what a dump" joke. I was nervous and cramped before, but now I was nervous, cramped, and intimidated.

I was told I'd be filming with a group of comedians, watching clips and providing commentary. Then I found out that these "other" comedians included some actual legends who had starred in huge movies, long-running TV shows, and Broadway. I was surrounded by greats. *Um, why am I here again?* Cue The Muppets singing "One of These Things (Is Not Like The Others)." I told myself I was probably just there as a space filler. Most of the comedians in this room were straight-up famous, and I am a nobody. So I could probably lay low, make two jokes, and leave without destroying my career and dignity. For a moment, the panic that had been coursing through my body lessened a bit. The panic, which, if I didn't know any better, was starting to feel less like nerves and more like period cramps. But there was no way I could be having period cramps, because I was on the pill and I was at Bill's mansion.

Just then, a character actress that I worshiped walked into the room. This woman, as far as I'm concerned, is one of the best character comedians on the planet and an inspiration. I took a deep breath and tapped her on the shoulder. Just as she turned, I heard a guy behind me say, "Amy? Amy Albert? I didn't know you would be here!" I spun around to see a middle-aged man grinning at me. I returned the smile, but my face gave away the fact that I had no idea who this guy was. His expression changed. "Hiiiiiiiii!" I said a little too enthusiastically. He wasn't buying it. "You don't remember me, do you?" he replied flatly. My mind started to race. *Do I owe him money? Did he see my boobs once? Did I black out and get catfished?* My face got hot, and those cramps that could not be "those" cramps flared up again. I said, with a voice barely louder than a whisper, "Jeez, I'm so sorry! I recognize you, but can't place your name." The man crossed his arms and bellowed, "Wow! If a pretty girl can't remember my name, then I won't be reminding her of it!" Then he stomped off. All eyeballs, including those of the famous, on me. The "that can't be my period" cramps seized violently, and sweat gathered in my armpits. After what felt like four days, one of the famous comedians broke the tension by yelling, "Thanks buddy, make this weirder!" I was mortified. I'm pretty sure this is not how people lay low.

Cal, who'd witnessed that shit show from across the room, waved me over. He could see the anguish on my face, and he quietly told me the name of the freakshow who just yelled at me in a room filled with my idols. We'll call him Wesley, and it turns out I *did* know him. Several years before, Wesley and I had been part of a short-lived improv company and had performed a few shows together. He acted like he gave me a kidney or something. Cal also informed me that Wesley was the executive producer (meaning he was paying for this production thanks to an inheritance) for the documentary and that I needed to apologize. Wait, *I* had to apologize? It's absurd in hindsight, but at this very moment I truly felt like I had blown it. So if apologizing would smooth it over and make this day less horrifying, fine. Wesley accepted my "apology," and a crew member alerted me that the filming was about to start.

Embarrassed and full of "non-period" ubercramps, I sat in the far-back, dark corner next to people way more successful than me. *Thank God. I really am just a seat filler.*

The screening began, and a cameraman moved around the space filming people's reactions. Once in a while, the director would pause a scene to ask the well-known actors and comedians questions like "What did you think about George's delivery there?" or "How important is timing for bits like these?" The answers were always poignant and articulated with great care. I laughed along at the appropriate moments and nodded in agreement during others. The knots in my stomach loosened for a second. Then the Martha Raye segments started. Amongst her bevy of talents, Martha Raye was a superb physical comedian. She was excellent at acting "drunk" in scenes, which is really hard to pull off well. One of the main reasons I was even chosen to participate in this film is because my character, Delilah Dix, is always drunk. Over-the-top falling down, losing her underpants at a parade, and waking up in a Tijuana bath house type of drunk. I took a lot of pride in performing as her, but I never once put any real thought into how to act drunk. And even if I did, it's almost impossible to describe. On cue, "Amy, your character, Delilah Dix, is a drunk, right? So you would know better than anybody, how do you play drunk successfully?"

I felt my face grow hot again, and those damn cramps pulsed. "I…well, it's always a good idea to not actually be drunk!" I said, hoping that would suffice as an answer. The group chuckled politely, but didn't turn back around. Cal made a gesture to expand on what I meant. Like, this is the question that only I can answer. Sweat was pooling in my bra. I waited for my brain to come up with the brilliant anecdote I was searching for, when my mouth decided for me: "Sad grace! You…have to have…sad grace." The group stared at me in silence with confused expressions, and Cal gave me a puzzled look. SAD. GRACE?! Wtf does that even mean? I shrunk back in my seat, completely embarrassed and sweaty, and prayed for a meteor to crash through the ceiling and take me out.

My cramping was now internal flogging. The AD called for a ten-minute break. I darted into the closest bathroom right outside of the screening room. I closed the door and locked it, and slid all the way to the floor. I immediately noticed two things. The first being that Bill's bathroom was as big or bigger than my entire apartment. The shiny golden-hued garbage can sitting under the Italian marble sink looked like it cost more than anything I'd ever owned. Then the second thing came into focus. Sitting on the imported tile floor with my legs gently splayed and the skirt of my dress hiked up to my thighs, something caught my eye. It was red. Blood red. Oh my God! My breath quickened as I yanked my dress up more. My eyes fell upon the homicide that had just happened in my underwear. No. Was this…hysterical menses or am I actually dying of embarrassment?!

The mess in my knickers was epic. There was dry, rust-colored blood covering the entire front of my panties, and it was stuck in a few places, so I had to gently peel it off my bikini line slowly so I wouldn't accidentally also give myself a waxing. The inside of the underwear was a whole other bag of gross. Period blood was pooled in the crotch of my drawers. I stared at it for a second and thought, okay, was I shot or something and am in shock? How could I not have noticed this was happening?

A PA knocked on the door. Ten-minute break over. I frantically attempted to clean up the blood that was creeping down my legs and took off my now-soaked underwear. I seriously felt like I understood what crime scene clean-up crews dealt with when they had a huge massacre on their hands. It seemed like there was period blood in places it should never be allowed to explore.

This period had evolved into an exclamation point. A period that, by the way, had no business being there for two more weeks! I hadn't brought a tampon or anything with me. Fortunately, I always carried an extra pair of underpants, which is due to years of living in New York City during humid summers resulting in damp panties and sweaty butt outlines on subway benches.

I wrapped the underwear into a toilet paper beehive and shoved it down to the bottom of the golden trash can. I threw on the fresh pair, piled a wad of paper into the crotch, and prayed that I hadn't left a Rorschach test image in period on the seat I'd been on during the screening. I walked slowly back to the back row and spent the following two hours hovering an inch above my seat. We cut, and I ran. I slumped into my rental car and cried all the way to the airport.

Fast forward eight years. I get a call from Cal. The film is coming out! It will be having a ton of screenings, things are moving forward, and…I was cut out of the film. The bits I had filmed previously didn't make sense in the final edit, and I'm sure "sad grace" didn't help. When I think back on that day now, I laugh instead of shiver and hop in the shower. The day I didn't get my big break, but did bury my bloody underpants in a golden garbage can in a mansion.

TECH SUPPORT

Technology, like your period, isn't always predictable. But like your period, technology is full of benefits! It can provide more info on your health and wellness, and it can help you feel like you're not alone in your menstruation journey. Jot down your tech faves on the next page.

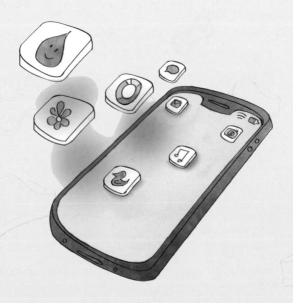

SOCIAL MEDIA

The periods hashtag on any social media platform will take you to profiles of menstruators and allies alike. Which ones have you followed?

_____   _____

_____   _____

_____   _____

WEBSITES

Several organizations are out there fighting against period poverty. Do an internet search to find ones near you and write down the ones you want to get involved with below.

_____   _____

_____   _____

_____   _____

ADDITIONAL RESOURCES

What other tech resources have you found helpful for your period?

_____   _____

_____   _____

_____   _____

"SIZE DOES MATTER"

By Renee Gauthier

There's something college girls and adult women all over the world tell themselves and each other to soothe their situations when they are found with a small penis in their lives.

"Size doesn't matter!" Typically followed by, "It's not the size of the boat, it's the motion of the ocean." Then everyone laughs and clinks their glasses of Chardonnay as the screaming silence of what they know the truth is…lingers.

Now, in my life…whenever someone says, "Size doesn't matter"…I first and foremost think of tampons. I promise there's a reason.

I have always been a little shy when it comes to talking about feminine topics, from tampons and periods to sex and penis size. I can trace it back to a moment when I was fourteen. 'Twas the first year of my menstruation.

It was the beginning of the school year, and I got my period on my birthday! The gift of womanhood also came with a full B cup of boobs, so all in all it was a good year.

I remember my friends getting their periods and hearing stories about their mothers celebrating their womanhood. I envisioned slow motion–style montages of them and their moms just buying tampons, pads with wings, and period pain meds. But I have never even seen feminine products in my house, so I figured my mom didn't get her period so she wouldn't care much. I was wrong. I told her, and she started to well up and took me to buy pads with wings. There was nothing else magical, but she was a single mom with four kids so I get it.

I cherished those pads because I was scared of tampons. I didn't think I was ready, until one day I had to use one during cheerleading season and I saw the light! So freeing, and if I had a horse, I could totally ride one! But I only would use the Light tampons. It was tiny, and in my brain, so was my experience of having anything in my body, so I thought it was the right thing to do.

One afternoon my Aunt Debbie was over, and she was not shy about much. Sidebar: she was married into the family and eventually married out if you know what I'm sayin'. Anyway, she yelled out…"Does someone have a tampon?" I was literally the only person in the room. So I told her that I did but they might be too small. She stared at me and said, "Why do you think I have a big vagina? Because I have had sex? Because I had a baby? Size doesn't matter!" I just stared at her, embarrassed that I even said anything while she continued to go off on a rant. She took one of my precious Light flow tampons and later bled through her pants.

From that point on, I knew I was right about the Lights. And as years went on and my periods evolved… I still look at every box of tampons and think of Debbie. Mostly I think about how she shouldn't ever be allowed to talk to young girls about their periods. I guess what I am trying to say is…I think size *DOES* matter, and I'm proud to be sometimes a Light, a Regular, a Super, and, on occasion, a SUPER DUPER DUPER. And I love that about me and my period.

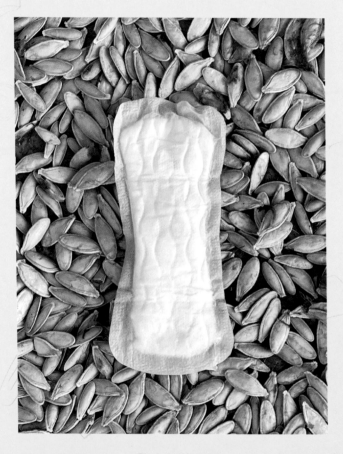

Photo by Neno

YOGA WHILE BLEEDING

SUKHASANA

Okay, time to cross my legs and breathe in. Is that…
am I getting my period? What day is it? Oh God, I
gotta breathe out. Breathe in. Maybe I can mentally
focus on delaying my period. Breathe out. Just gotta
really focus. Breathe in. Oh, it's definitely coming,
breathe in, breathe out, it'll be okay, breathe out.

HALF MOON

Standing up is good. Check the mat. Okay. Nothing
there. Fab. Oh, instructor sees me not focused. Be
focused. And stretch to the right. And center. Still
nothing. Stretch left. And back to uh-oh. Definitely
getting my period. What day is it?!

BACK BEND TO HANDS TO FEET

Just sticking my bloody behind in some other practitioner's face. I'm wearing black pants. And they're also
bent over. So maybe they won't notice.

AWKWARD POSE

Yeah, awkward is exactly right.

EAGLE POSE

Oh, squishy. Great.

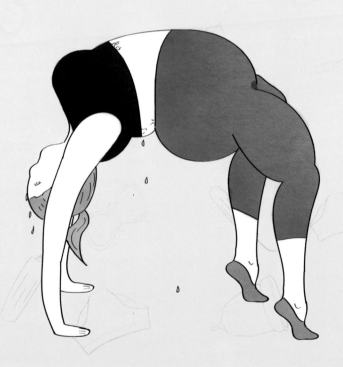

WARRIOR II

You know what? That's right! I *AM* a warrior! I'm a strong, fierce, powerful, BLEEDING WARRIOR! I SHALL BLEED FREE! I SHALL BE A REPRESENTATION OF WHAT MENSTRUATORS CAN BE OH GOD I WISH I HAD A TAMPON IN RIGHT NOW!!!

TREE POSE

Okay, this one isn't so bad… Maybe it stopped.

PLANK — CHATURANGA — DOWNWARD FACING DOG

Let's just get into a flow. Flow. FLOW. AUNT FLO! Damnit. There it is.

CHILD'S POSE

Well, sticking my literally bloody butt out again, but damn, this feels so good. At least I'm stretching out the incoming cramps while there's the outpouring of blood…

SAVASANA

Mmmmmm. I'm so glad I brought my own mat.

HOW TO
TALK TO
EACH OTHER
ABOUT YOUR
PERIOD...

OPENLY
AND
HONESTLY

"THE LIFE CYCLE"

By Bekah Tripp

She is told that it will come. She is told it is natural. She is told that every woman gets it. "Did the neighbor, Barb, get it?"

…"Yes, even Barb"

It comes. It is a tidal wave. It is a homicide in cotton underpants.

The years pass. It does not let up. It is relentless.

She thinks, "This is a bait and switch."

She thinks labeling this as "special" is false advertising.

She learns new words and phrases: "endometriosis," "laparoscopy," "cyst," "Code Red," "PMS," "miscarriage"…and several more.

Aunt Flo is a relative to half the population, and she gets around.

It causes many embarrassing mortifying moments throughout her formative years. She gets used to it, but she never greets it happily.

Except…

Some random months, when it comes, it is relief; it is a reprieve.

She gets pregnant, on purpose, and it goes away. Thank, Goddess.

It comes back.

And it's worse.

It worked out while it was away. It brings the pain on a whole new level. She puts up with it. The dudette abides.

She ages. It comes and goes. It is inconstant (better than incontinent…but that happens too). It finally leaves. But it does not leave quietly.

It brings weight…and leaves it. It brings sweat… and drenches her. It sucks up the moisture… everywhere.

Its friends slowly fall away. Ever. So. Slowly.

And then. She is alone. She is empty. Finally.

She begins anew.

She is slower. She is older.

But she is free.

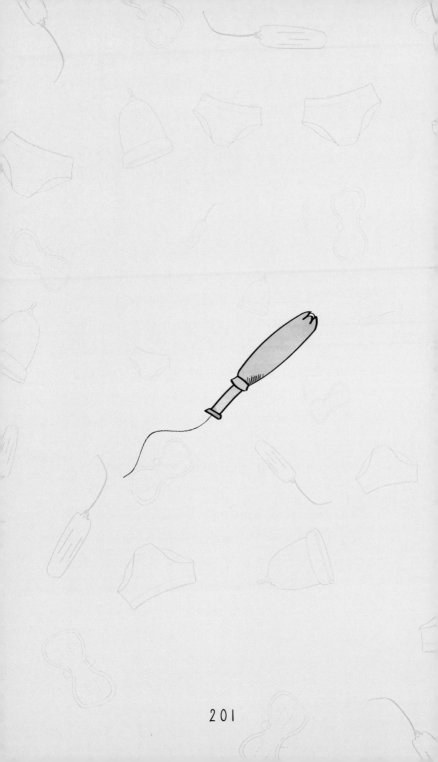

201

"DAY 2"

By Artemis Pebdani

Once, I was fancy and went to Greece with a friend. And that was cool. Until we had to travel back to the United States. It so happened that my flight out of Greece was delayed by half an hour, and that was just enough time for me to miss my connecting flight out of Istanbul, Turkey. At the ticket counter, I was assured that everything would be fine—they were kind enough to hold my luggage, whether I liked it or not, and I would be put promptly on the next flight taking off in a short twenty-four hours.

So, okay, yeah, that was an inconvenience. Also an inconvenience: my period had just started. Like, right as I was flying out of Greece. Now, as a lady person who had been around long enough to know some things, I knew my period was supposed to come around that time, so I wasn't totally unprepared. I had my menstrual cup in my purse, just in case.

***An important sidenote here about the menstrual cup: man, do I wish that shit worked for me. I mean, it *kinda* does. On the first day only. But something happens on Day 2 where (and I'm just guessing here) my insides take on an entirely different shape, making the menstrual blood miss the cup entirely and project around the sides to shoot right out of my vagina, and that seems to make a bigger mess than if I wasn't using anything at all. (Is that a thing? Lady insides changing shape during menstruation? Anatomists, I'm listening.) Same situation on Day 3: big ol' splatter mess. Then, from Day 4 on, there's usually not enough blood to lubricate an easy removal of the silicone apparatus, so it's just a drawn out twenty-minute Brechtian silent-scream-dance while I try to work against the physics of vacuums and suction. That part is, to say the least, not very sanitary. And before you DM me, yes, I've tried different brands in both sizes (standard lady and previously pregnant/over thirty-five lady). Trust me: the insides morphing/projectile perioding theory is the only thing that makes sense.

But that shouldn't be a problem here. It's only the first day. The menstrual cup is gonna carry me for now. I've got money. I'm in Atatürk International Airport, one of the largest airports in the world, a mega-hub of crisscrossing flights, transporting thousands of passengers a day—a sizeable percentage of whom, I would venture to guess, are women who menstruate. I'll just buy an overpriced pack of tampons and post up at a boozeless bar until this slight inconvenience is over.

Oh, wait—"no," you say? No tampons for sale in this very not small airport? Or pads either? How about NOT A SINGLE FEMININE HYGIENE PRODUCT IN THE ENTIRETY OF THE WHOLE. DAMN. PLACE. Not in a bathroom. Not at the newsstands, and somehow not in any of the six Chanel stores or fourteen duty-free perfume depots—nary a tampon or pad to be found. ANYWHERE.

…Is it because traveling women don't get their periods? Or they should just be discreet enough to be fully prepared to quietly take care of the offensive bodily function that is THE NECESSITY FOR HUMAN EXISTENCE without forcing everyone to have to look at related products on blatant display at a sales counter? After all, actually seeing a pad or a tampon for sale would make men have to think of… periods. Blech! Can you imagine? Helping women be comfortable while they willy-nilly bleed out of their *ahem* *parts*—an act that just so happens to be the very SOURCE OF LIFE—the reason you and I and everyone since always is here?!

  ***Important sidenote #2: I know, for a fact, this can't be summed up as a "Muslim thing." I come from a Muslim family. I have it on good authority that there are indeed feminine hygiene products for sale in the Muslim world. *This* is a "dudes being in charge" thing. *This is the tunnel vision of patriarchy.* Now, I've seen a similar occurrence (but on a much lesser scale) at more than one gas station here in the States. Where the only feminine hygiene products for sale are pads that double as neck pillows and tampons that are so big, they somehow have two applicators. Those are obviously "dudes being in charge" cases as well. But after this experience, I've got to give those gas stations a little bit of credit, because this…this is outright ex*emption*??

  To say I was enraged would be an understatement.

  Gosh, what's the term for "insidious misogyny"?

  Oh right—INSIDIOUS MISOGYNY.

  Eff you. Eff you, that dude who runs that airport. Eff you, that dude in charge of supplying those airport stores and bathrooms. At best, you don't think about women. At worst, you do, and your childish disgust for women exhibiting this (I cannot stress this point enough) REQUIREMENT FOR THE INITIAL AND CONTINUED PRESENCE OF THE SPECIES supersedes their comfort and necessity. *Eff you, that dude.* And if by chance that dude is a woman…he's not. Eff that dude.

Okay—I'll bring it back down and not harp on the issue anymore. If you're reading this, I'm gonna bet we're on the same side here anyway. Or at least I hope so.

Here's what really matters: that was just Day 1. Also, if you're reading this, then you're probably quite aware of this fun fact—it's on Day 2 of your period that shit gets real.

So, here I am on Shit Gets Real Day, finally catching that connecting flight back to Los Angeles. As soon as I board the plane, I do that asshole move where I unload all of my crap in my seat and elbows-out my way to the bathroom. This is, after all, an ocean-crossing flight, so the plane should be more "readily equipped," and by that I mean I was looking for one of those airplane sanitary pads. In case you didn't know, lots of airplanes actually do have sanitary pads available in the bathrooms. To prevent theft (I assume), they come in the size of an adult forearm, but I'll be damned if it's not a welcomed sight when you need it. Surprise, surprise, this flight…did not have pads available in their bathrooms.

What did I do? Well, I did what women and junior high girls have done since the beginning of time. I fashioned my own Build-A-Pad from the only tools available to me: one-ply airplane toilet tissue and paper towels (emphasis on the "paper"). For those of you that somehow haven't had to do this and are curious, you're basically looking at a burrito recipe. The paper towel acts as the tortilla with loads of toilet paper folded back and forth for the filling. Honestly, you really don't need the paper towel tortilla. If you've got even kind of enough thigh, the layered toilet tissue filling will stay in place on its own (sort of) and do the same, equally mediocre job. The tortilla is mostly just wishful thinking in the form of Martha Stewart flair. For real, I don't know what possibly makes up the technology of today's pads to be so thin and amazingly absorbent. It can't be good for the environment. It's probably not good for your body, but boy, is it effective. As opposed to *actual* toilet tissue and *actual* paper towels—which don't really do much.

With my crotch craft in place, I fought my way back up the aisles to my row and over my row mates to my window seat. See, I like the window seat, because I prefer to chill and pass out, and I don't have to worry about people bugging me to get up, and *I* won't bug people to get up because I'm passed out, remember? But not that day. Not on Day 2.

As soon as I would feel my tissue burrito getting overly saturated, I would bug the lady and gentleman next to me to get up and let me through to the bathroom to construct a fresh booster seat. Then I'd bug them to get up again and let me back into my corner of shame. And I kept doing that—about every two hours for the duration of the *fourteen-hour* flight. I did that even down to the "tray tables up" announcement. And you guessed it, they were pretty pissed off by then, because that announcement is the final announcement where they say, "Buckle up and be done doing shit folks, because we're getting ready to land." And if you're a rule follower at all, you are not happy about having to get up after that directive. Who knows? The successful landing of the plane may be in jeopardy. But I did what I had to do. I asked them to spit caution in the face and let me get up and go to the bathroom one final time. After a non-verbal "are you fucking kidding me" in various degrees from both of them, I finally just laid it out. "Look, I'm on the second day of my period, and I was stuck in a

Turkish airport for a day with no feminine hygiene products to be found. Either help me out and get up, or I'm gonna bleed all over the place here, and that's gonna be on your head."

The guy was decent enough to fall back, and I assume the lady was probably on board by the time she heard "second day of my period."

Hmph. I *guess* we can say this story had a happy ending? I didn't bleed all over the place, so there's that. I *did* make a long-ass, uncomfortable flight even more uncomfortable for two people aside from myself. That's not so happy.

You know, there are all these feelings about what a crappy thing our periods are (I *know* I'm not alone here). Like, it's just this giant drag and a burden to most women that we've had to deal with throughout all of known time. Shoot, it's nearly always a bummer for me, and I've had to live with it for *literal dozens of years*. But I can't help but think it would suck at least a weeeee bit less if it wasn't this huge shameful secret. If there was some societal accommodation or at least an out-loud acknowledgement that nearly half of the population deals with menstruating for a significant portion of their lives, and mentioning it wasn't met with discomfort or revulsion. Ah, fuck it—

The insidious misogyny!! To disregard and, more-over, be *repulsed* by periods—

The PREREQUISITE TO REQUISITES?! Oh, eff you, dude. Seriously. Eff. You.

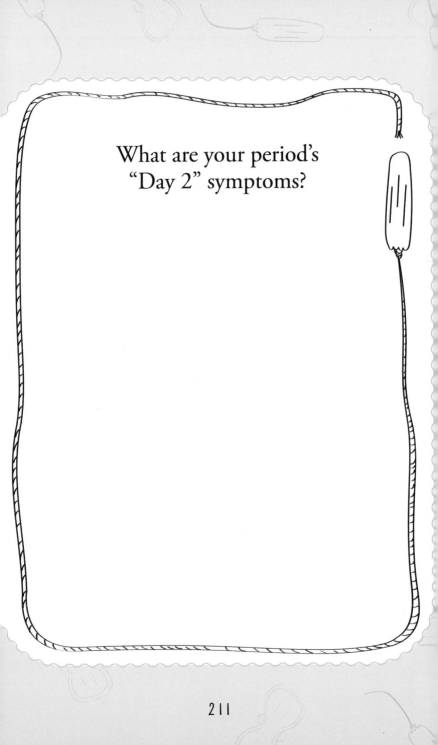

What are your period's
"Day 2" symptoms?

"WE ARE NOT TOTALLY FINE"

By Alisha Gaddis

"Like my body is expanding and ripping in shreds while simultaneously being stabbed by a knife as the pain shoots down my legs, making them radiate with pain, and the fatigue is so heavy I can't pick up my arms."

That's exactly what I told my husband when he asked how my cramps were today.

I bet he is SUPER glad he asked.

But that's what my period always feels like for me.

IT IS FINE! I AM FINE! WE ARE ALL FINE!

I can do everything during my menstrual cycle. Right?!?

Yes, I can totally sit on this Zoom and fake smile through the agony. Sure! I can lead this meeting with half-open eyes, still heavy from lack of sleep, unable to get comfortable at night. Yes, I can totally take the kid to lyrical class and talk to the other parents while I wince with pain. Absolutely! I can wear this dress to that event and not feel like a stuffed sausage walking bloated through life. YES, I can pretend like it doesn't hurt.

I am totally fine.

We are totally fine.

We are told to be fine.

We are not fine.

I had absolutely zero idea that the amount of debilitating pain I felt every four to ten weeks was "not normal." (Oh yeah—my period is just as unpredictable as the clearance rack at a designer discount store and just as savage as the people who shop there).

My mom was this way, too. One year, she canceled Christmas because of "stomach pains" (decades later I would learn the truth about her quiet suffering).

I suffered in silence, because I was taught to suffer in silence, as I am sure my grandma did, and her mama, and their mothers before them.

Why are we taught to act like we are not bleeding out of our bodies and in pain?

Who are we covering for?

When my dam breaks and the flood hits, I am literally knocked out with the rushing waters.

Middle school—I'd hide tampons in my bookbag. Experience cramps so bad I would cry in the stalls, alone. Bleed through cheerleading bloomers during the game. Stuff wads of harsh toilet paper in my Hanes underwear after I bled through my winged pad. Constantly fear toxic shock syndrome. Never talk to my VERY best friends about it. Never.

High school—Almost fall asleep in AP Calculus from low iron. Snap at my Lit teacher when my pain was so high that I almost turned into *Lord of the Flies* on her. Bleed through my jeans during my first dates at the movie theater. Bury, deep in our half bath trashcan, soaked underwear. Never talk to my mom about it. NEVER.

Never allowed to miss a class.

Never allowed to complain.

Never questioning the amount of ibuprofen I put into my young body to make it stop.

College—Freshman year. I was struck by such pain in my right ovary that I vomited into the toilet and passed out on the floor. My boyfriend at the time freaked the F out. There I was on the floor, bleeding from my head and my vagina. Poor guy—I was so much more than he bargained for.

I woke up in the hospital looking at a different manchild who must have JUST graduated from my college. He had a thumb ring on under his plastic gloves and a puka shell necklace sitting on his oddly tanned neck.

He leaned in closely to me and said that he liked my toenail polish.

Totally normal for a doctor.

As I sat naked from the waist down, legs spread akimbo, he and his jewelry examined my nether regions.

Someone brought in charts and x-rays.

"Wow! One of your ovarian cysts was the size of a giant golf ball and it burst! I'd only heard about this in med school. Cool."

I had no idea what he was talking about.

He winked at me and held the x-rays to the light.

I stared at the screen. My ovaries now looked like a juicy cluster of grapes, ripe for the picking. Tons of fluid-filled baubles ready to POP open and cause excruciating pain.

Cool, cool, cool.

This led to birth control, which led to weight gain, which led to taking myself off birth control, which led to heavier periods, which led to a fear of all things vagina, which led to more pain, which led to more cysts bursting and more suffering in silence.

This was not normal.

Today, I have a child—who I had to fight against my cysts to make.

Today, I have an IUD—which makes the pain and bleeding less but does not make it go away.

Today, I choose to not suffer silently—which has liberated my heart and my flow.

But it still hurts and isn't fun and I don't like it.

Not cool.

Today, as I sit with a heating pad on my lap, adult acne on my nose, and radiating pain down my thighs, I write this hoping my daughter will seek solace, will get help, and we can break the cycle of suffering in silence.

For her grandma, and for her grandmother's daughter, and herself, and maybe her own child one day.

Because even if we aren't fine, we can be not fine, together.

LAUGH UNTIL YOU CRY PERIOD JOKES!

With Kristine Kimmel & Jessie Gaskell

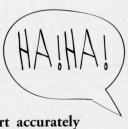

What is the average age women start accurately tracking their periods?

55-65

What's the best age to start your period?

The Jurassic

If buying tampons makes them queasy...

Wait until they find out you can eat your placenta!

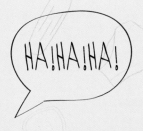

THE NIGHT OF THE BIG DANCE

Ask a friend to fill in each blank prompt according to their mood. Then read the whole thing out loud and expect uproarious laughter!

Tonight is finally the night. I am going to the big

DANCE! I've waited _____ months for this! I cannot
(NUMBER)

wait to _____ there with Shawnta! All our hopes and
(VERB)

_____ are coming true.
(NOUN)

My dress is so _____. I feel like a _____! This
(ADJECTIVE)   (PROPER PRONOUN)

is going to be everything I dreamed of!

Let me take one last look in the _____.
(NOUN)

Holy crap! Is that period blood on my dress!!?!

NOOOOOOOO!!!! _____ !
(EXPLETIVE)

I feel _____.
       (EMOTION)

This is a disaster of epic _____.
                    (NOUN)

Deep breaths. Remember my mantra: "Right now it's

like _____. Soon it will be _____."
     (NOUN)   (FOOD)

It's fine. Tie-dye has been all the rage lately.

Maybe everyone will think this is intentional?

Maybe I will set a new trend?

Or maybe I will curl up and _____ .
                           (VERB)

"Shawnta? You're here! What? You think I look

_____? And you love my _____?
(ADJECTIVE)   (CLOTHING ITEM)

"OMG thanks! Yes. It was all totally on purpose."

Whew! I am so _____.
              (ADJECTIVE)

Let's go to the dance and party through the period!

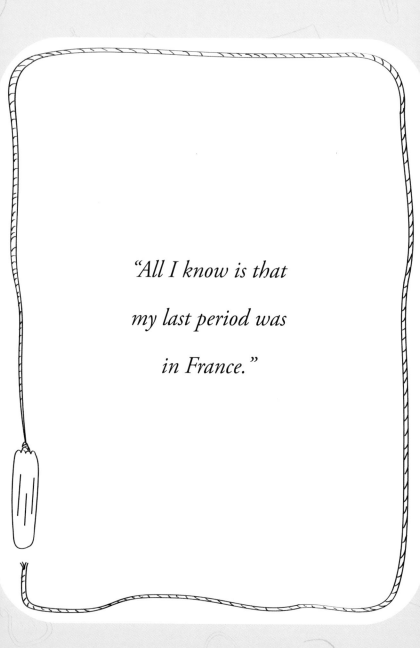

"All I know is that

my last period was

in France."

MENOPAUSE MAMIS

We interviewed a group of menopausal women to get their thoughts on their periods and the last leg of the period journey. Here are their best responses. Names have been changed at the request of the mamis.

Q: What was your relationship with your period?

"My relationship with my period was sort of like having a bad friend that showed up when you least expected it." —Diana

"I got my period when I was ten years old, almost eleven. In those days there were only pads and tampons. The pads were huge and bulky. You had to clip them on a belt-like thing with clip-ons and underwear. Not only was it uncomfortable, but there were many accidents. I never liked my period." —Cher

"[My mom] sat me down and said, 'You are going to get this menstrual flow every month. You are to wear this sanitary napkin. Take an extra to school. Do not let any boys touch your private parts. You are now a señorita.' I was totally stunned." —Dolly

Q: What did you know about menopause before, and did you research it at all?

"All I had heard about menopause was about the hot flashes, the intermittent periods, headaches, the sweats at night. I did not research anything on menopause; I accepted it as part of a cycle that women go through and it was 'normal.'" —Gloria

"I knew nothing about menopause since it started invading my life quite early—when I was in my forties! But I did consult my doctor on why I felt like I was experiencing 'heat waves' that came and went all the time. After consultations, biopsies, and blood work, he concluded, 'You ran out of gas my dear, you entered menopause!'" —Diana

"I didn't do any research on menopause. All I know is that my last period was in France." —Dolly

Q: What's the difference between perimenopause and full-on menopause?

"Gee, I still don't know what perimenopause is." —Dolly

"In my case, the only difference was my period stopped completely with full menopause, and the hot flashes were more frequent and stronger." —Gloria

"I was never in perimenopause! When I consulted my doctor, I was told I was in full menopause! Horrible night sweats. When everyone was freezing, I wanted to take off all my clothes, and would have hot flashes that would drive you bananas." —Diana

"I began getting headaches and one time, I thought I was having heart issues, but I was told this was probably perimenopausal symptoms. After a few years, I noticed I was sometimes missing my period, but it would then come back. That went on for a few years, and then, all of a sudden, I realized that my period hadn't been around for a few months." —Celine

"Perimenopause is like a roller coaster—you just never know which way it's going to go, and you don't know it's coming. With menopause, you know you're done and this is it…. In my case, perimenopause was way worse than menopause. It lasted almost ten years!" —Cher

Q: Anything fun about menopause?

"FUN? Oh yeah, YOU STOP HAVING YOUR PERIOD!! And this is nice!" —Diana

"No need for birth control ::crying laughing emoji::" —Celine

"There's a certain freedom that comes with it in conjunction with an empty nest. I think it makes you feel young in your mind, not necessarily your body." —Cher

"There's nothing funny about menopause. 'Suck it up, old ladies.'" —Dolly

Q: Final thoughts?

"There are many menopause babies, sooo just make sure that when the period stops, that it is due to menopause and you're not, nine months later, holding a bundle of joy!" —Gloria

JOURNAL PROMPTS

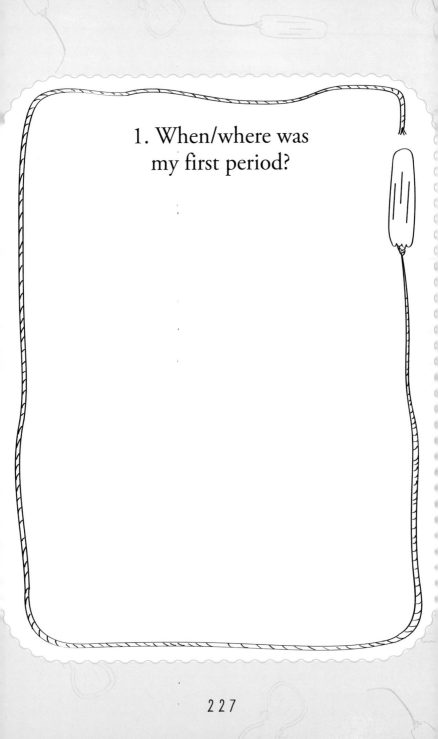

1. When/where was my first period?

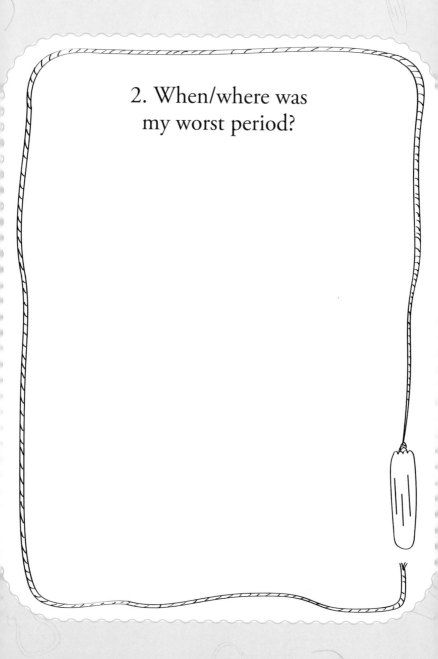

2. When/where was
my worst period?

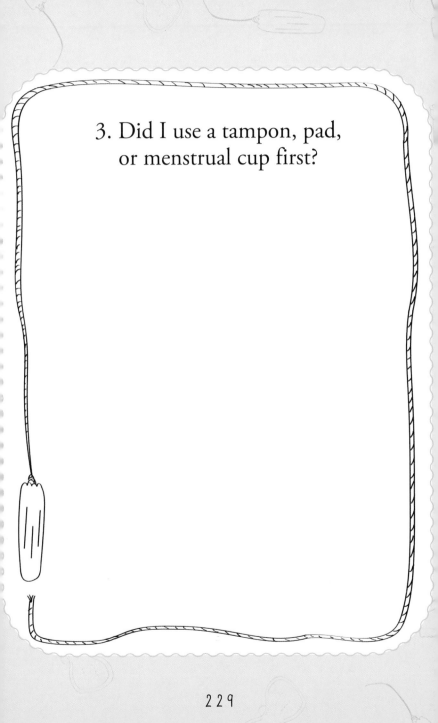

3. Did I use a tampon, pad,
or menstrual cup first?

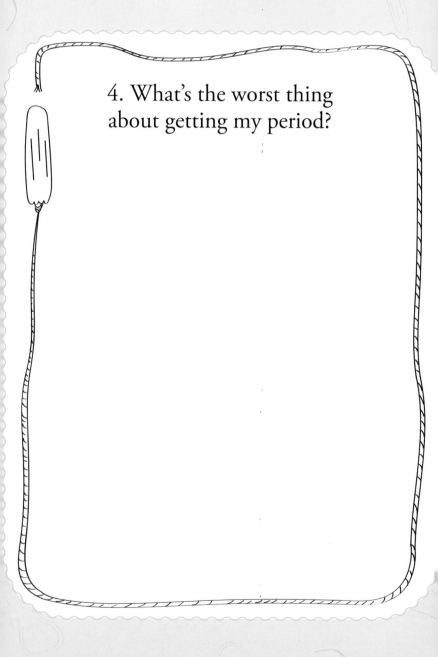

4. What's the worst thing about getting my period?

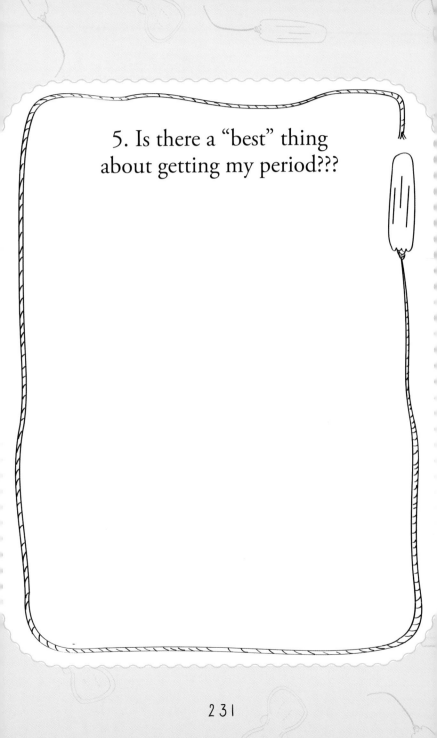

5. Is there a "best" thing about getting my period???

6. Who do I feel comfortable discussing all the bloody details with? Why?

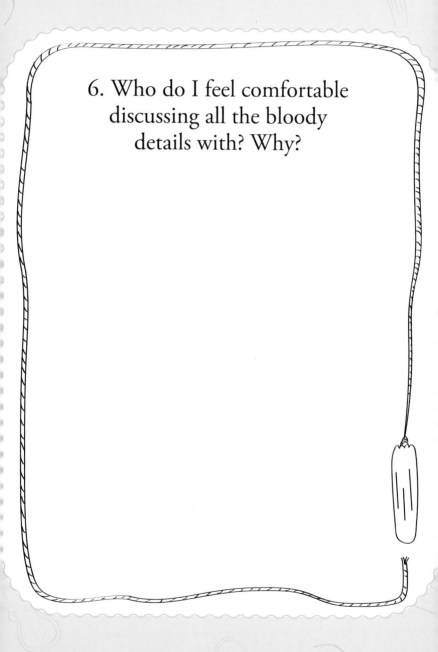

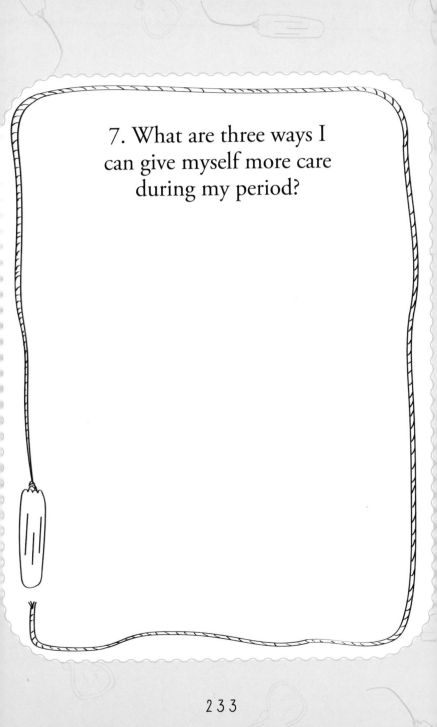

7. What are three ways I can give myself more care during my period?

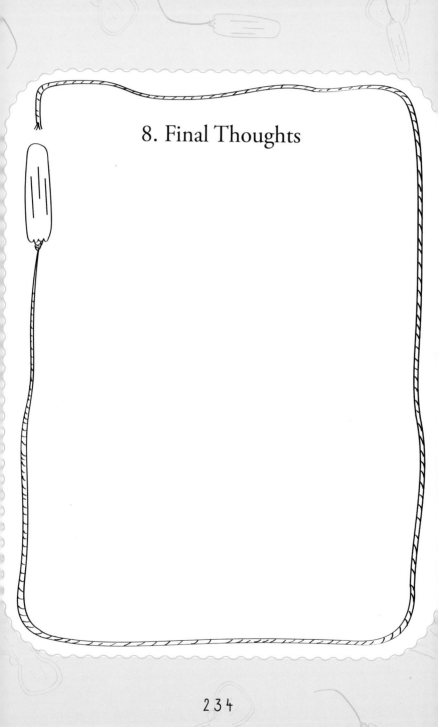

8. Final Thoughts

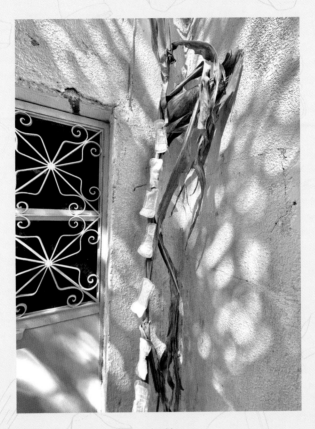

Photo by Neno

ABOUT THE AUTHORS

Alisha Gaddis is an Emmy Award–winning actor and multi–Latin Grammy Award winner in Los Angeles. She is a graduate of New York University Tisch School of the Arts.

Alisha has published multiple books to critical acclaim. As a filmmaker, she is currently in development on her first feature with her writing partner and has sold an animated series for Latin America. She is a National Endowment for the Arts Grant recipient. As executive producer and co-creator of a hit PBS show, Alisha garnered multiple Emmy nominations and one win.

Gaddis was named one of the funniest upcoming female comics by *Entertainment Weekly* (hopefully it translated into this book)!

Gaddis adventures with her husband and young daughter, Indiana Maven. She's now explained menstrual cycles to her six-year-old way too many times.

Steph Garcia hosted the storytelling podcast, *That's My Story Period* for Campfire Media, all about menstruation.

She's an alumnus of the National Hispanic Media Coalition TV writing program and has written for a variety of television programming.

She is also a mom who hopes that one day her kids will be both embarrassed and delighted by this book.

Desireé Nash is thrilled, as a longtime menstruator, to have her illustrations published for the first time in this book.

Desireé is also a writer, animator, and independent filmmaker. She has written and directed three short films: *Dumped* (an Official Selection of the 2017 Women Texas Film Festival), *Sort of Friends,* and *Brain on Drugs* (an Official Selection of the 2019 Bad Film Fest). Her feature screenplay was awarded Best Feature Screenplay at the LA Under the Stars Film Festival. She is also currently working on her first indie animated short film.

Desireé is from Corpus Christi, TX, and now lives in Los Angeles, CA, with her hopes and dreams.

CONTRIBUTORS
IN ORDER OF APPEARANCE:

Martina Papinchak

Carissa Kosta

Kate Tellers

Shelley Friedman

Hannah Sterling

Liz Kocan

Lorraine DeGraffenreidt

Mazzy Miziker

Sarah Monsoon

Irene (Neno) Diaz

Levi Yates

Lori Elberg

Kristine Kimmel

Jessie Gaskell

Kay Kaanapu

Katharine Davis Reich

Jessica Shein

Emily Churchill

Susie Mendoza

Ilana Cohn Sullivan

Seneca Dykes

Laurissa Gold

Malynda Hale

Bekah Tripp

Katy Kassler

Meg Swertlow

Brennon Dixson

Amanda Hirsch

Jessica Glassberg

Dani Adaliz

Grace Kestler

Madeleine Hernandez

Zurie Cobb

Amy Albert

Renee Gauthier

Artemis Pebdani

The Menopause Mamis

SPECIAL THANKS

Alisha and Steph would like to thank our agent, Sara Camilli, who was a continual and vocal advocate for this book. You never gave up in finding it a home. We're so deeply grateful for you.

We would also like to thank all the wonderful and talented contributors who gave their creative energies towards this book. The book is only great because of the sum of its parts.

To the Post Hill Press team, especially Debra Englander, Heather King, and Madeline Sturgeon, thank you so much for believing in this book.

Finally, thank you Desireé Nash for the incredible illustrations you've crafted throughout the book. (Dez! You made such amazing work! We love it! We love you!)

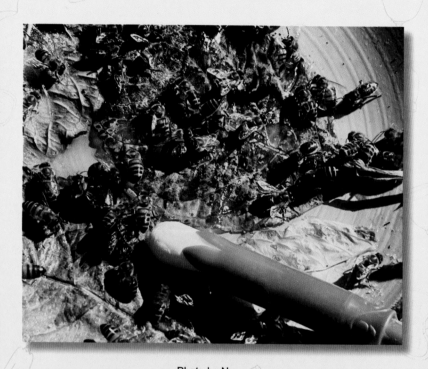

Photo by Neno

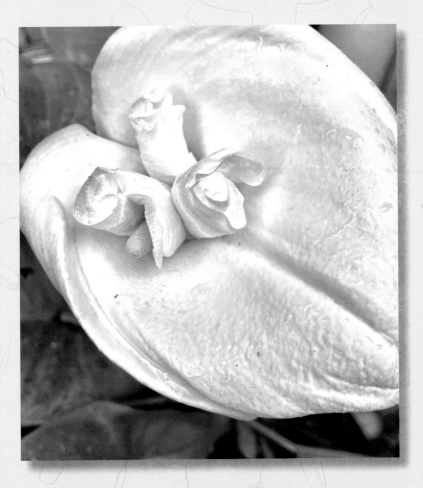

Photo by Neno

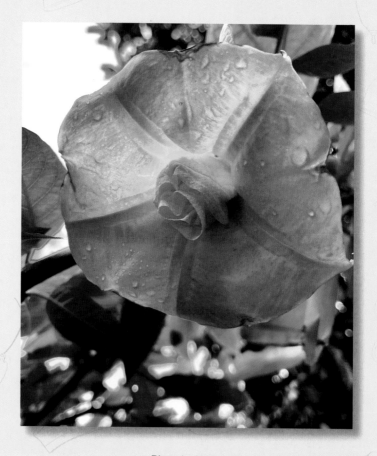

Photo by Neno

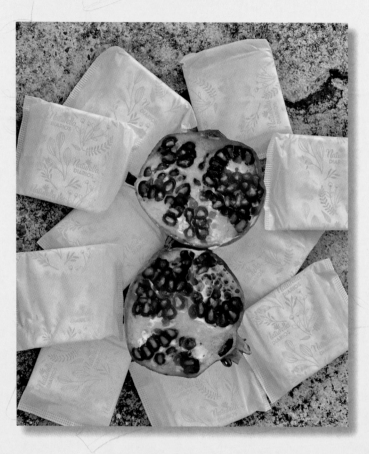

Photo by Neno

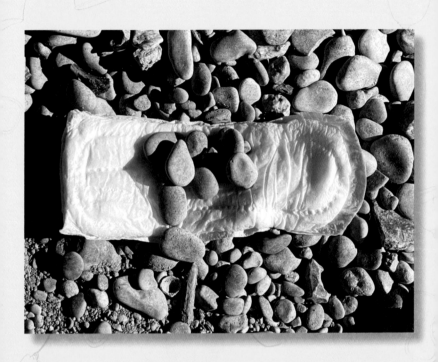

Photo by Neno

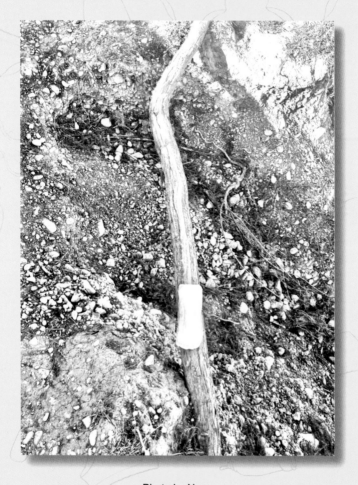

Photo by Neno

ANSWER KEY

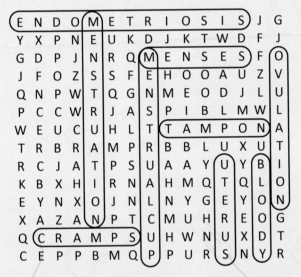

UTERUS   MENSTRUAL CUP   MENSES
TAMPON   MENSTRUATION   CRAMPS
BLOODY   ENDOMETRIOSIS   OVULATION

REFERENCES

Ally Corner:

https://www.huffpost.com/entry/congress-fighting-over-tampons_n_5b36516fe4b0f3c221a04984

Marathon Bleeding:

https://www.cosmopolitan.com/health-fitness/q-and-a/a44392/free-bleeding-marathoner-kiran-gandhi/

Periods of the World:

Scotland –
https://www.bbc.com/news/uk-scotland-scotland-politics-51629880

China –
https://www.npr.org/sections/goatsandsoda/2016/08/17/490121285/a-swimmers-period-comment-breaks-taboos-in-sports-and-in-china

Space –

https://www.theatlantic.com/health/archive/
2016/04/menstruating-in-space/479229/

Ireland –

https://www.nytimes.com/2021/04/20/world/
europe/ireland-period-products-lidl.html

Sweden –

http://www.mtv.com/news/2355116/dancing-
tampons-crush-period-stigma/

Antarctica –

https://womensadventureexpo.co.uk/well-what-
do-i-do-with-a-tampon-in-antarctica/